ENT Practicals
MADE EASY®

ENT Practicals MADE EASY®

Sujatha S
MBBS DLO DNB MNAMS PhD
Associate Professor of ENT
Government Medical College
Thiruvananthapuram, Kerala, India

Foreword
Viswanathan N

JAYPEE *The Health Sciences Publisher*
New Delhi | London | Philadelphia | Panama

Jaypee Brothers Medical Publishers (P) Ltd.

Headquarters

Jaypee Brothers Medical Publishers (P) Ltd.
4838/24, Ansari Road, Daryaganj
New Delhi 110 002, India
Phone: +91-11-43574357
Fax: +91-11-43574314
E-mail: jaypee@jaypeebrothers.com

Overseas Offices

J.P. Medical Ltd.
83, Victoria Street, London
SW1H 0HW (UK)
Phone: +44 20 3170 8910
Fax: +44 (0)20 3008 6180
E-mail: info@jpmedpub.com

Jaypee-Highlights Medical Publishers Inc.
City of Knowledge, Bld. 237, Clayton
Panama City, Panama
Phone: +1 507-301-0496
Fax: +1 507-301-0499
E-mail: cservice@jphmedical.com

Jaypee Medical Inc.
325 Chestnut Street
Suite 412, Philadelphia, PA 19106, USA
Phone: +1 267-519-9789
E-mail: jpmed.us@gmail.com

Jaypee Brothers Medical Publishers (P) Ltd.
17/1-B, Babar Road, Block-B, Shaymali
Mohammadpur, Dhaka-1207
Bangladesh
Mobile: +08801912003485
E-mail: jaypeedhaka@gmail.com

Jaypee Brothers Medical Publishers (P) Ltd.
Bhotahity, Kathmandu, Nepal
Phone: +977-9741283608
E-mail: kathmandu@jaypeebrothers.com

Website: www.jaypeebrothers.com
Website: www.jaypeedigital.com

Inquiries for bulk sales may be solicited at: jaypee@jaypeebrothers.com

ENT Practicals Made Easy®

First Edition: **2016**

ISBN: 978-93-5250-113-7

Printed at Rajkamal Electric Press, Plot No. 2, Phase-IV, Kundli, Haryana.

Dedicated to

All my teachers, who guided me to learn;
and to all my students, who inspired me to teach

Foreword

The era is witnessing a profuse influx of information and technology. As these spread to each and every part of life, the medical education also cannot stand apart. The beauty and efficiency of a systematic patient approach may get extinct in the near future with the present overdependence on technology. A well-taken medical history and systematic examination of the patient, often, leaves little room for mistakes. The importance of history taking and a proper examination of the patient should never be diluted by diffusion of technology.

It is in this context the book *ENT Practicals Made Easy*® by Sujatha S is so important and timely. Her long service as faculty in medical colleges as undergraduate and postgraduate teacher has helped her to bring out this book in an outstanding manner. She guides in a systematic way with an umbrella of logical mind. It is a pleasant and palatable approach which will definitely be an user-friendly one for the medical students.

I have had the pleasure and honor of associating with Sujatha for a long time. She is a well-known academician in the field of otorhinolaryngology. Her own techniques of endoscopic surgeries and facial cosmetic surgeries are remarkable. She is one among the best clinicians I have worked with. She is a very good teacher and thirsty for knowledge and that is testified by this beautiful book. I am proud that I could associate with a person like Sujatha who believes and practices the fundamental principles of clinical examination.

Viswanathan N
Professor of ENT and former Superintendent
Government Medical College
Thiruvananthapuram, Kerala, India

Preface

The surgical subspecialty, ENT, includes a vast array of topics, lessons and ideas; but only a small portion is required to be studied by the undergraduate medical students. ENT is perhaps the simplest and one of the most interesting specialties at that level. Practical examinations, especially objective structured clinical examination (OSCE) and viva need very precise and accurate answers to the questions. Even though many of the medical students are thorough with the subject matter, the majority of them are not able to answer the questions of the teachers in a satisfying manner. I too have faced this tricky situation during my student career, and I found that the dilemma continues even with the present generation of students.

This book is the result of my endless endeavors to find a solution to this problem. It contains the way to discern patient history, how to examine a patient and also presents a variety of questions commonly asked in practical examinations, together with answers in the section of X-ray, Instrument and OSCE. I have tried to include several pictures and to make content simple, so that even a mediocre student can understand the subject matter. A student who does a thorough reading of this book can reasonably expect a first class in the practical examinations and go on to become a seasoned professional in the future.

Sujatha S

Acknowledgments

I am indebted to ...

My father, late Panayur C Sankarankutty, who was a constant source of my inspiration and support to all my endeavors, and who wished this dream of mine to come true.

My teacher, Professor S Sasikumaran Nair, who taught me what ENT means.

Professor N Viswanathan, Professor K Sasikumar and Professor J Mohan, who have always helped, trusted and supported me.

Professor L Vijayalakshmi, Vice Principal and Convenor, CHEP Medical College, Thiruvananthapuram, Kerala, India, for guiding me to walk in the ideal path of learning and teaching.

I am thankful to Shri Jitendar P Vij (Group Chairman), Mr Ankit Vij (Group President), Mr Tarun Duneja (Director–Publishing) and Mr KK Raman (Production Manager) of M/s Jaypee Brothers Medical Publishers (P) Ltd, New Delhi, India.

Contents

Introduction

Dear students, ENT is a specialty that you can never avoid in your clinical postings and also in practicing years. Sure that you all will become consultants in near future. Most of the cases in pediatrics, medicine, gynecology, surgery or in general practice includes those of ear, nose or throat. I told this only to emphasize the need of learning ENT not only to pass examination, but its importance in your entire career.

As beginners in learning the art of medicine, the importance of good history taking is beyond doubt. As you have completed your medicine and general surgery postings, you may be knowing the basic principles of this. But ear, nose and throat are different from all other parts of the body. They are hidden areas and you cannot examine them as you examine abdomen or limbs. Small size and anatomical inaccessibility make it difficult for the teacher to demonstrate to all students at a time. That is why, we need good illumination and special instruments for examining ENT.

CHAPTER 1

History Taking

Even in this era of sophisticated investigations, good history taking remains as an essential skill and need for an accurate diagnosis.

Name: Most beautiful word to ones ear is his own name. Try to call your patient by his/her name.

Age: Congenital anomalies commonly seen in early childhood. Tonsil and adenoid hypertrophy is seen in children. Nasopharyngeal angiofibroma is seen in puberty. Presbycusis happen in old age. Malignancies seen in older age group, though no age is immune to it.

Sex: Nasopharyngeal angiofibroma seen in males. Malignancies of head and neck except postcricoid malignancy is common in males. Atrophic rhinitis and otosclerosis is common in females.

Occupation: Occupation helps to know the socioeconomic status, in reaching a diagnosis and in planning treatment. Voice disorders due to chronic laryngitis, vocal nodule, vocal polyp, gastroesophageal reflex disease, etc. are mostly seen in school teachers, lawyers, singers or preachers. Sinonasal malignancies are more in woodworkers and those in metal and petroleum refineries.

Residence: Documentation of residence helps in research purpose and follow-up of patient. Rhinosporidiosis is common along coastal areas.

PRESENTING COMPLAINTS

Common presenting complaints are as follows:

- *Ear:* Earache (otalgia), ear discharge (otorrhea), hearing loss (deafness), headache, fever, swelling in and around ear, itching, giddiness, ringing in ear (tinnitus), deviation of angle of mouth, inability to close the eyes.
- *Nose:* Nasal discharge (rhinorrhea), nasal block, facial pain and headache, bleeding from within the nose (epistaxis), smell disturbances, postnasal drip, speech defect, sneezing, cresting, itching nose, epiphora, snoring, deformity of nose.
- *Larynx and pharynx:* Change in voice, difficulty in breathing, noisy breathing (stridor), cough, sorethroat, foreign body sensation in the throat, mouth breathing, dysphagia (difficulty in swallowing), odynophagia (painful swallowing), swelling neck.

All these should be written in chronological order. If multiple complaints of same duration, write according to severity.

HISTORY OF PRESENTING COMPLAINTS

Narrate this in patient's own language. Avoid medical terms as far as possible. Negative history may be helpful at times.

Details of each presenting complaint should be asked.

Earache (Otalgia)

Pain in the ear may be due to lesions in the ear itself or due to diseases in areas having same dermatomal innervation (Referred Otalgia).

- Duration
- Constant or intermittent/is it aggravated/relieved by anything? (Pain of external otitis may be aggravated by chewing, opening mouth or by touching pinna)

- Character—whether it is dull aching, stabbing, pricking type
- Severity—pain is very severe in furuncle ear, acute otitis media and perichondritis of pinna. Mild in uncomplicated chronic suppurative otitis media, wax, etc.
- Whether unilateral or bilateral.

Otorrhea

- *Duration:* Acute, chronic or acute exacerbation of chronic disease.
- *Scanty/Profuse:* Discharge is usually scanty in dermatitis of external canal and chronic suppurative otitis media atticoantral disease (CSOM-AAD). In tubotympanic disease (CSOM-TTD) discharge is profuse.
- *Constant/Intermittent:* If intermittent, relation with upper respiratory infection or water entry to ear should be asked. Such a history is usually associated with CSOM-TTD.
- Character of discharge:
  - *Watery (serous):* CSF otorrhea, diffuse otitis externa, early stage of acute otitis media.
  - *Mucoid:* Discharge is sticky in nature. Produced by mucus glands present in middle ear. Seen in ASOM/CSOM. It shows that discharge is coming from middle ear through a perforation of tympanic membrane.
  - *Mucopurulent:* Colored tenacious ear discharge. Seen in ASOM/CSOM (active).
  - *Purulent:* Thick tenacious discharge. Common in external otitis with furuncle, otomycosis, cholesteatoma, etc. This purulent discharge usually signifies an underlying bone eroding process in middle ear.
  - *Bloodstained (serosanguinous):* Seen in ear trauma, malignancy, barotrauma, hemangioma, glomus jugulare tumor, granulation ear, etc.

Hearing Loss

Ask about:

- *Onset:* Whether onset is sudden or gradual.
- *Duration:* Congenital deafness may be due to genetic causes or prenatal/perinatal maternal factors like intake of drugs or infections. Deafness of recent onset is due to trauma, infections, vascular, metabolic, etc.
- Severity
- *Laterality:* Whether bilateral/unilateral.
- *Nature of deafness:* Improvement during periods of discharge seen in active stage of CSOM. Paracusis Willisii (improvement of hearing in noisy surroundings) seen in otosclerosis. Recruitment present in cochlear lesions. Fluctuating deafness seen in secretory otitis media and Meniere's disease.

Giddiness

This symptom should be asked in detail as this term is most often interpreted wrongly by the patient. Sense of unsteadiness is termed as giddiness, but vertigo is a hallucination of movement of body or surrounding. It is a subjective feeling of imbalance. This sensation is very unpleasant and patient may vomit during attacks of vertigo. Try to know the exact feeling the patient is having. Find out whether it is true vertigo or a syncopial attack in which patient gets a black out or just a giddiness. Note any history of preceding upper respiratory infection. Ask how and when it started, duration of each attack, frequency of each attack, association with other complaints like nausea, vomiting, tinnitus, hearing loss, visual problems, seizures, history of migrainous attacks, any drug intake, trauma and thyroid medication.

Tinnitus

Ringing sensation in the ear. It can be subjective (heard only by the patient) or objective (heard by other persons also).

Here also enquire about mode of onset, duration, whether unilateral/bilateral, severity, periodicity and associated symptoms.

Nasal Block

- *Duration:* Helps to say whether disease is acute/chronic.
- *Whether unilateral/bilateral:* Unilateral nasal block is common in deviated nasal septum, foreign body nose, antrochoanal polyp, etc. Bilateral nasal block seen in ethmoid polyps, allergic rhinitis or septal hematoma.
- Whether constant or intermittent.
- Whether progressive in nature or not.

Nasal Discharge

- Unilateral or bilateral.
- *Types of discharge:*
  - Watery discharge seen in early stages of common cold, vasomotor rhinitis and CSF rhinorrea.
  - Mucoid discharge is common in allergic rhinitis.
  - Purulent in atrophic rhinitis, FB nose, furunculosis.
  - Bloodstained in malignancy, FB, nonhealing granuloma, nasal myiasis, etc.
  - Mucopurulent discharge is seen in infective rhinitis, sinusitis, malignancy, etc.
- *Amount:* Scanty/Moderate/Copious.

Facial Pain and Headache

Ask

- *How it started:* Spontaneously/induced by something like trauma
- How long the pain last?
- Any aggravating/relieving factors
- Any associated symptoms like visual disturbances (aura of migraine) nausea, vomiting, giddiness, associated numbness/ toothache

- Any diurnal variation (change with time of day/night)
- Does associated with restricted/painful neck movements.

Headache of each sinusitis have typical characters:

- *Frontal sinusitis:* Headache of frontal sinusitis is usually located in frontal and superciliary area. Pain aggravates on looking down. Headache is more when patient wakes up in the morning, lasts for few hours and relieves by evening. This is called *office headache* as pain present during office hours. This is due the gravity dependent drainage of frontal sinus.
- *Maxillary sinusitis:* Pain more on upper jaw, teeth and spread over cheek. Usually dull aching type more towards evening. Pain more on stooping or coughing.
- *Ethmoid sinusitis:* Pain more marked in children. Movement of eye will be painful and associated with lid edema. Pain localized over nasal bridge and inner canthus behind the eye.
- *Sphenoid sinusitis:* Headache is experienced in the vertex or occiput. Severe cases are associated with visual problems.

Epistaxis

Confirm whether fresh blood, clotted blood or bloodstained discharge.

- Enquire about amount of blood loss
- History of trauma causing epistaxis
- Intake of any drugs like anticoagulants
- Bleeding from any other sites
- History of similar episodes in the past should be asked.

Disturbances of Smell

- *Anosmia:* Total loss of smell (seen in head injury, intracranial mass lesions or functional)
- *Hyposmia:* Reduced sense of smell (rhinitis, nasalpolyp, nasal allergy)

- *Parosmia:* Altered sense of smell (allergic rhinitis)
- *Cacosmia:* Any smell is experienced as fowl (chronic sinusitis).

Postnasal Drip

Defined as waterfall like whitish discharge seen in posterior wall of oropharynx. Patient will tell as excessive discharge coming from behind the nose causing various pharyngeal symptoms. Postnasal drip occurs more in allergic and infective diseases of nose, nasopharynx (adenoids and Thornwald's disease, bursitis) or paranasal sinuses (sinusitis).

Change in Voice

Nose and paranasal sinus give timber to our voice. In nasal mass and in rhinitis, there will be a nasal twang of voice. Mass in the nasopharynx cause rhinolalia clausa. Cleft lip, cleft palate and postadenoidectomy patients speak in rhinolalia aperta.

Sneezing

Occasional sneezing is a normal nasal reflex. Excessive sneezing is seen in allergic rhinitis.

Pain in the Throat (Sore Throat)

Enquire whether pain or discomfort, present at rest or during chewing and swallowing, duration, progressive or not, constant/ intermittent, localized/spread to surrounding area, associated symptoms like fever, change in voice, swelling neck, etc.

Difficulty in Swallowing (Dysphagia)

Ask whether swallowing difficulty is due to pain on swallowing (Odynophagia) or food does not pass down below or both.

Hoarseness is usually due to diseases in the laryngopharynx.

Neck Swellings

Can be enlargement of thyroid or cervical lymph nodes or salivary gland swellings.

Like this positive and negative history of each presenting complaint should be asked and noted down.

HISTORY OF PAST ILLNESS

Ask about

- Similar complaints in the past
- History of diabetes mellitus, hypertension, bronchial asthma, pulmonary tuberculosis
- History of *exanthematous fevers* (influenza, scarlet fever, viral pneumonia, measles, etc. can lead to *acute necrotizing otitis media*)
- History of any surgeries in the past (if present enquire done under general or local anesthesia, duration of hospital stay, any intraoperative/postoperative complications)
- Allergy to drugs (aspirin hypersensitivity seen in ethmoid polyp)
- History of allergic rhinitis.

PERSONAL HISTORY

- Bowel/bladder habits
- Sleep/appetite
- *Addictions:* Important in malignancies. In smokers, calculate the number of pack years (number of packets per day multiplied by years of use).

FAMILY HISTORY

- Similar complaints in the family (otosclerosis run in families, so also sensoryneural hearing loss)

- *History of overcrowding:* Overcrowding is defined as "two persons of opposite sex having age above 9 years forced to live in same room, because of a situation in which more people are living within a single dwelling than there is space for, so that movement is restricted, privacy secluded, hygiene impossible, rest and sleep difficult"
- Socioeconomic status (calculate per capita income or ask APL/BPL ration card)
- History of diabetes mellitus, hypertension, bronchial asthma in the family.

MENSTRUAL HISTORY IN FEMALES

Thyroid disorders are usually associated with menstrual disturbances.

TREATMENT HISTORY

Drugs like salicylates, aminoglycosides, quinine and cytotoxic drugs can cause deafness. Tinnitus is the first important symptom of salicylate poisoning. Patients taking ototoxic drugs may also get vertigo. Glossitis, stomatitis, etc. are seen after chemoradiation. History of treatment for hypo/hyperthyroidism should be asked as it is usually associated with complaints of voice and throat. Drugs like warfarin and anticoagulants can cause epistaxis.

CHAPTER 2

ENT Examination

Before doing examination of ear, nose and throat, it is essential to do *examination of patient in general* starting from head to foot. Start with build and nourishment (ill/moderale/well-built) of patient.

Note: Gait, pallor, edema, icterus, cyanosis, jaundice and generalized lymphadenopathy. Examination of skin for dermatitis, rash, pyoderma, etc. are important in cases of nasal allergy and ethmoid polyposis.

Next is examination of ENT. Before going to that it is essential to know about the instruments used for examining ear, nose and oral cavity given in detail under section of Instruments in ENT.

- *Source of light is Bull's eye lamp:* It is kept behind the left shoulder of the patient at the level of his left ear. It has a convex lens and contain 100 W bulb.
- *Head mirror (Macenzy's):* Concave mirror with outer diameter of 9 cm and that of central aperture is 2 cm. Focal length of mirror is 25 cm.
- *Spirit lamp:* Used to warm laryngeal or postnasal mirror.
- *Gloves* for palpating oral cavity, oropharynx and nasopharynx.
- *Xylocaine spray* to anesthetize oropharynx to abolish gag reflex.
- *Ear speculum of different sizes:* For better visualization of external auditory canal and tympanic membrane. *Toynbee, Hartmann, Politzer* and *Tumarkin* are names of different types

of specula. *The largest speculum which can be conveniently inserted in the ear canal should be used.*

- *Otoscope* with pneumatic speculum. Magnification power × 2.
- *Jobson-Horne's probe and ring curette:* For removal of wax and debris of ear canal.
- *Tuning forks (Gardiner-Browne tuning fork)* of 512 Hz frequency is commonly used. Other frequencies available are 128, 256, 1024 Hz, etc.
- *Nasal speculum:* The size of the speculum is selected according to the age of the patient and size of the nostril.
- *St Clair Thompson postnasal mirror:* Size 1 or 2 is ideal.
- *Nasal endoscopes:* Rigid endoscopes (30° and 0°) or flexible nasopharyngolaryngoscopes.
- *Lack's tongue depressor:* For examining oral cavity and oropharynx. Also used to do cold spatula test.
- *Laryngeal mirror:* For indirect laryngoscopic examination, various sizes from 6 to 10 are available.

EXAMINATION OF EAR

Look for any abnormalities. If no change from normal write as normal.

1. Pinna

Look for change in size, shape, position.

- Size—microtia, macrotia
- Shape and position—abnormalities of contour seen in cauliflower ear, Singapore ear, etc. Pinna stands out prominently and the postaural groove gets obliterated in furunculosis. Pinna is displaced downwards and outwards in mastoiditis with subperiosteal abscess.
- Redness—furuncle, abscess.
- Swelling—hematoma, abscess, sebaceous cyst.

- Scar—Trauma or previous ear surgery. William Wilde's postaural incision scar is common after mastoid surgery.
- Hairy tragus and pinna along with earlobe crease found to be having in patients with coronary artery disease.

2. Preauricular Area

Look for preauricular sinus, cyst, appendage, tag, accessory tragii or lymphadenitis. If none of these present, write as normal.

3. Postaural Area

Postaural scar is noted after mastoid surgery and mastoid abscess after drainage. Lymphadenitis, cyst, etc. may also be present. Edema at the exit of mastoid emissary vein in the postaural area (Griesinger's sign) is seen lateral sinus thrombosis.

4. Tragal Sign

Presence of pain on pressing tragus or on moving the auricle is *positive tragal sign*. Seen in external otitis.

5. Mastoid Tenderness

Elicited by three finger test. Look for pain on pressing over Cymba concha, tip of mastoid or lateral surface of mastoid (nonhair bearing surface posterior to pinna). Never press simultaneously on these points. Of these three sites most reliable point is Cymba concha (**Fig. 2.1**) as it directly overlies mastoid antrum. Mastoid tenderness present in acute mastoiditis.

6. External Auditory Canal (EAC)

It is never a straight canal. It is S shaped canal of 24 mm length. Hair of cartilaginous part also prevents proper visualization of tympanic membrane. *So pinna is pulled upwards backwards and*

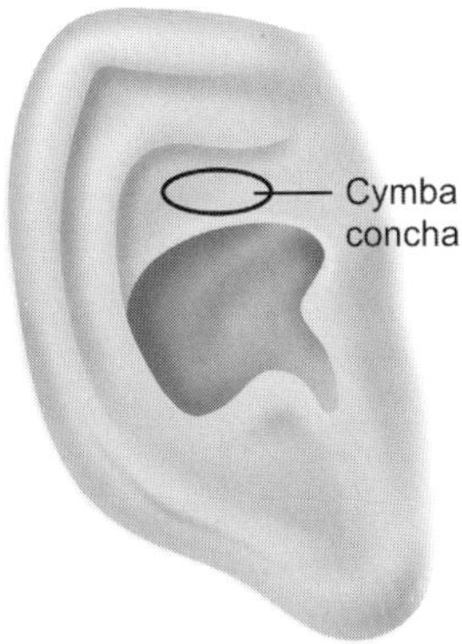

Fig. 2.1 Right pinna showing Cymba concha

laterally in adults, downwards, backwards and laterally in children to straighten the canal. If there is pus in the canal, it should be cleaned with cotton tipped applicator (dry mopping). Similarly, wax should be removed carefully to see tympanic membrane. Wax, debris, pus, polyp, furuncle, granulation, osteoma, etc. are likely to be seen in the canal. Sagging of posterosuperior canal wall is seen in acute mastoiditis.

Examination of Ear with Speculum

If EAC is narrow, or if presence of excessive hair in EAC, ear speculum is needed for proper visualization. Always use proper size ear speculum to avoid trauma to canal. Gently introduce into ear canal with rotating movements and pass just beyond the junction of bony and cartilaginous canal and membrane is examined.

7. Examination of Tympanic Membrane

Normal tympanic membrane (TM) is pearly white, semitransparent with cone of light in the anteroinferior quadrant (Pars tensa is

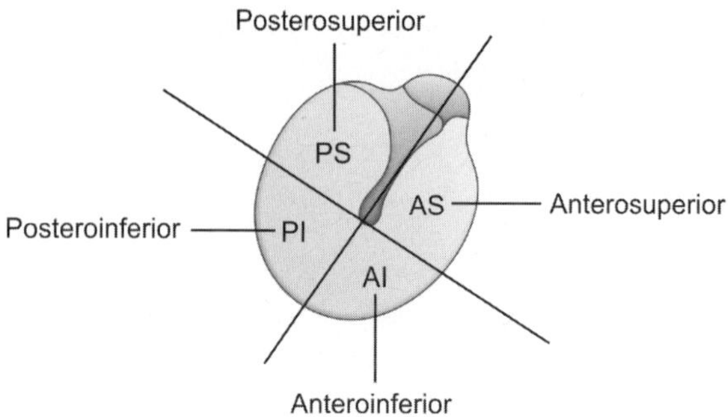

Fig. 2.2 Right TM divided into quadrants

divided into four quadrants by two imaginary lines; one parallel to handle of malleus and second horizontal line intersect it at the umbo) **(Fig. 2.2)**. Abnormalities of the membrane are noted with respect to the quadrants involved. Look for mobility of tympanic membrane, this is done by siegalization or by valsalva manoeuvre. While drawing normal tympanic membrane remember, it is oval in shape, handle of malleus is directed towards left in right TM and towards right in left TM and cone of light starts from tip of handle of malleus in the anteroinferior quadrant **(Fig. 2.3)**.

Normal Tympanic Membrane

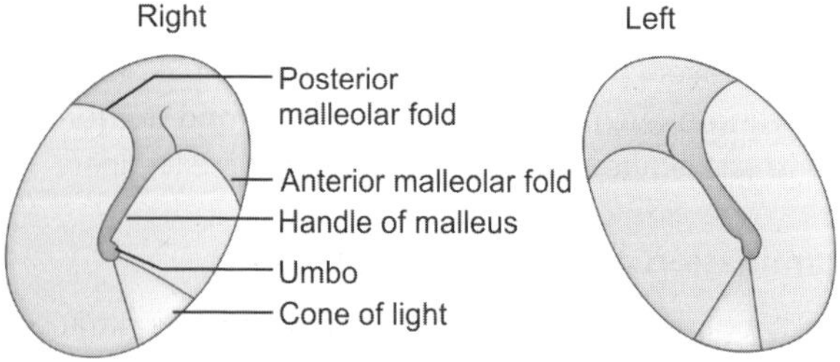

Fig. 2.3 Normal tympanic membrane

Abnormalities of Tympanic Membrane

Retraction

Features of retracted tympanic membrane are:

- Membrane is dull, lusterless.
- Absent or distorted cone of light.
- Foreshortening (apparent shortening) of handle of malleus.
- All landmarks (anterior and posterior malleolar folds, lateral process of malleus, annulus) become prominent.
- Mobility will be restricted.
  Because of all these, there will be mild conductive hearing loss.

Retracted membrane commonly seen in aero-otitis, secretory otitis media and adhesive otitis media.

Color

- Red—acute otitis media, bullous myringitis.
- *Flamingo pink reflex:* Active stage of otosclerosis.(Schwartze's sign).
- Blue color of membrane common due to blood in middle ear after trauma called *hemotympanum*.
- Chalky white patches are called *tympanosclerosis*.
- Waxy appearance seen in secretory otitis media.

Perforation

Look for type, size, shape, margins of perforation and status of middle ear mucosa:

- *Attic perforation **(Fig. 2.4)***: Perforation in Pars flaccida.
  - Indicates underlying cholesteatoma.
- *Central perforation **(Fig. 2.5)**:* Perforation in Pars tensa with remnants of tympanic membrane all around.
- *Marginal perforation* **(Fig. 2.6)** is perforation of tympanic membrane not covered by remnants of tympanic membrane

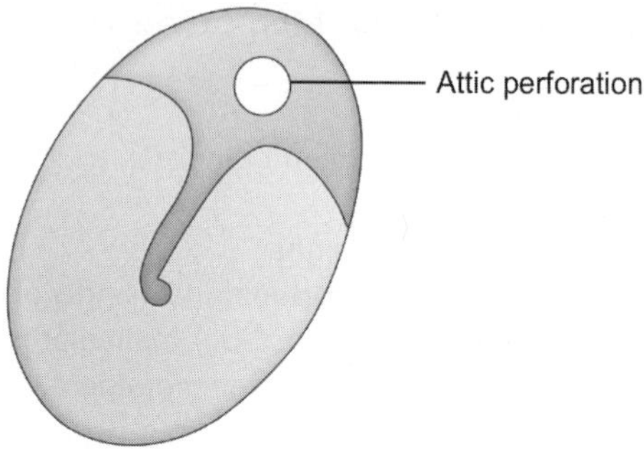

Fig. 2.4 Right TM showing attic perforation

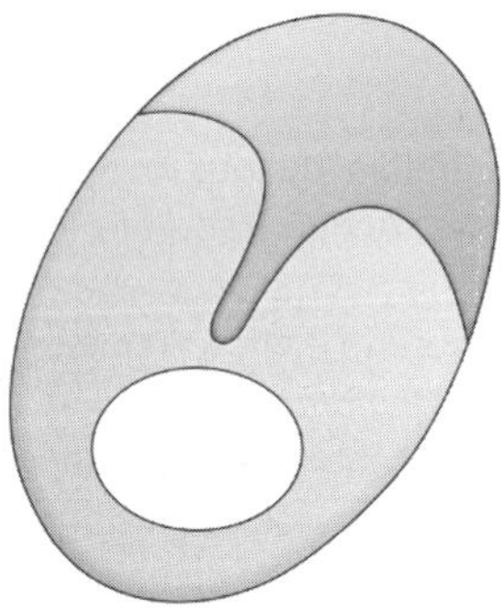

Fig. 2.5 Right TM showing central perforation

all-around so that exposing a part of annulus. It can be in Pars tensa or flaccida. It indicates unsafe ear.

- *Retraction pocket* ***(Fig. 2.7)***: Common site is in the postero-superior quadrant. Retraction pockets are marked with dotted lines.

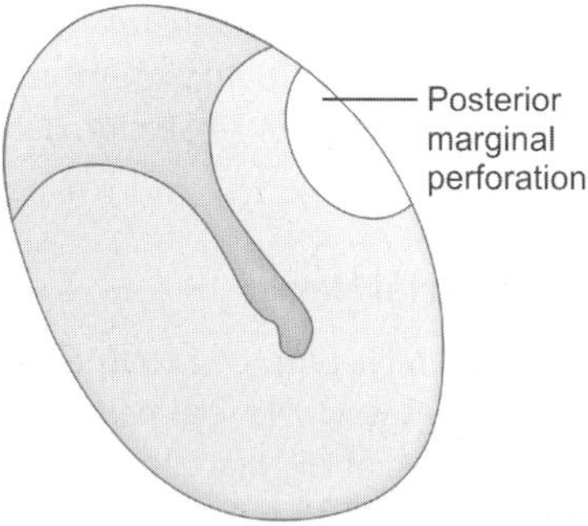

Fig. 2.6 Left TM showing posterior marginal perforation

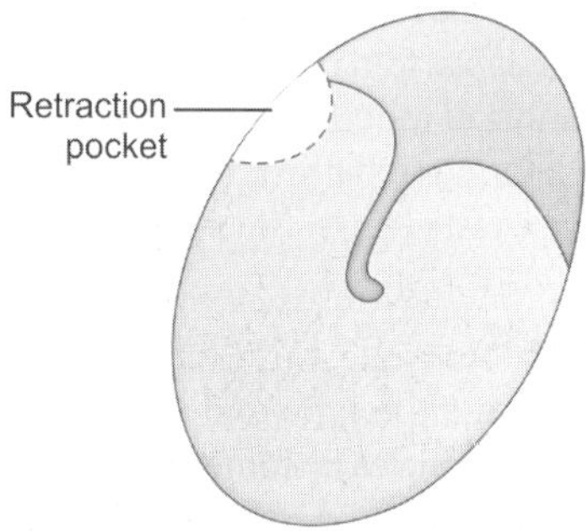

Fig. 2.7 Right TM showing posterosuperior retraction pocket

Points to Differentiate between Perforation and Retraction Pocket

- Margins are seen in perforation not in retraction pocket.
- Mobility is absent in perforation but present in retraction pocket except in adhesive otitis media.
- Middle ear mucosa seen in perforation not in retraction pocket.
- Handle of malleus more prominent in retraction. Usually, it is eroded in perforation.

Do a probing under microscope to confirm.

Assess the mobility of tympanic membrane by Valsalva maneuver (mobility best seen in posterior part of TM) or by Siegalization.

8. Examination of Facial Nerve

Lower motor neuron (LMN) type of facial nerve palsy is seen commonly with ear diseases. LMN facial palsy affects one side of face. Common clinical signs of LMN facial palsy are:

- Absence of wrinkling of forehead on the affected side
- Inability to close the upper eyelid. Eyeball rolls upward in attempted closure of eye. This protective mechanism is called *Bell's phenomenon* and this is *Bell's sign*.
- Absence of nasolabial fold on affected side.
- Deviation of angle of mouth to normal side.

There are other topographic tests for facial nerve like Schirmer's test, stapedial reflex, taste test, submandibular salivary flow test.

9. Tuning Fork Test

Tuning fork tests assess the type and amount of hearing loss a patient is having. Frequencies of commonly used tuning forks are 128 Hz, 256 Hz, 512 Hz and 1024 Hz. Of these, the most commonly used one is of 512 Hz due to the following four reasons:

1. This frequency comes in speech range (500–2000 Hz).
2. Overtones are less.
3. Optimum vibration sense.
4. Optimum decay time.

Parts of Tuning Fork (Fig. 2.8)

For vibrating a tuning fork, *ideal surface to strike is resilient and nonelastic surface like hard rubber.* It can also be activated by striking against any bony surface. Prong should be struck at a

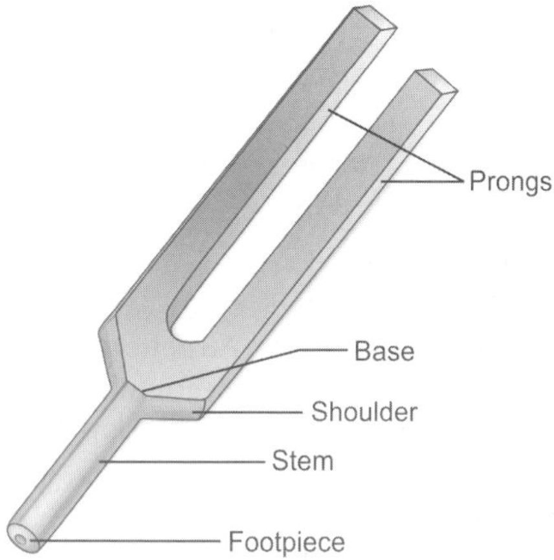

Fig. 2.8 Parts of tuning fork

point about one-third of the length from the free end to reduce overtones.

Routinely done tuning fork tests are:

Rinne Test

Air conduction (AC) and bone conduction (BC) of the test ear are compared. There are two ways of doing this test:

1. *Threshold comparison method:* Activate the tuning fork. Place its footpiece on the nonhair bearing skin immediately posterior and superior to external auditory canal. When the patient stops hearing place it in such a way that prongs vibrate against the ear in line with external canal at a distance of 2.5 cm.
2. *Loudness comparison method:* Activated tuning fork is kept alternatively over postaural area and in front of external auditory canal. Ask the patient which sound stops first. This is a better method because ear has the property of adaptation and patient will not hear, if kept continuously over the mastoid.

Table 2.1 Quantification of loss of hearing with Rinne's test

256 Hz	*512 Hz*	*1024 Hz*	*Interpretation*
Negative	Positive	Positive	Mild conductive hearing loss
Negative	Negative	Positive	Moderative chronic hearing loss
Negative	Negative	Negative	Severe chronic hearing loss

Interpretation of Rinne's Test

- *Rinne's positive:* Normal person. AC better than BC.
- *Reduced Rinne's positive:* Seen in sensorineural deafness.
- *Rinne's negative:* Seen in conductive deafness. BC better than AC.
- *False negative Rinne:* Seen in severe unilateral sensorineural deafness. BC is better because of contribution from other ear. This is avoided by masking the normal ear.
- *Rinne's test equal:* Minimal conductive deafness. AC = BC
- *Rinne's positive infinitely:* AC only, no BC. Seen in severe sensorineural deafness. Rinne's test can be used to find out the degree of hearing loss as in **Table 2.1**.

Weber Test

Vibrating tuning fork (footpiece) is kept either on the vertex, root of nose or on the upper incisor teeth. Ask the patient, where he hears the sound (at one ear/both ears).

Interpretation of this Test

- *Weber central:* Normal hearing.
- *Lateralized to diseased ear:* Conductive deafness.
- *Lateralized to better ear:* Sensorineural deafness.

Absolute Bone Conduction Test (ABC/Modified Schwaback's Test/Pomeroy's Test)

This test compares the absolute bone conduction of the patient with that of examiner, assuming that examiner's hearing is normal.

Activated tuning fork is held on the mastoid of the patient closing the external meatus firmly with tragus. Patient is asked to signal when he no longer hears the sound. Then transfer the tuning fork to the examiner's mastoid closing the external meatus.

- *ABC reduced:* Sensorineural loss. If the examiner still hears the vibration of the fork, when the patient has stopped hearing, then the bone conduction of the patient is reduced. This is seen in sensorineural deafness.
- *ABC normal:* If the examiner also does not hear the sound then test is regarded as normal. ABC is normal in conductive hearing loss (HL) as well.

  This test is absolute and cannot be prolonged.

Of these *Weber test is most sensitive*. Even 5–7 db airbone gap can be found out by this test. Rinne's test to become negative, need atleast 20–25 db airbone gap.

- Teal test, Stenger's test and Chimani-Moss test are done in suspected cases of nonorganic hearing loss (NOHL).
- Lewis test, Bing test and Gelle's test are special tests in otosclerosis.

Other tests for nonorganic hearing loss (NOHL) are:

- Erhard and Lombard tests are voice tests to diagnose NOHL
- Inconsistency of pure tone and speech audiometry
- Acoustic stapedial reflex
- Bekesy audiometry (type V wave)
- Brainstem evoked response audiometry.

10. Spontaneous Nystagmus

Nystagmus is involuntary rhythmic, regular and oscillatory movement of eyeball.

Method to elicit Nystagmus: It should be done in good light. Patient seated in front of examiner. Head is kept steady. Patient asked to follow the direction of fingertip of the examiner. Fingertip is moved horizontally and vertically in the field of vision of the patient not more than 30° from midline. Spontaneous involuntary rhythmic movements of eyeball is noted.

11. Fistula Test

Method: Pressure change is applied to ear canal either by alternatively compressing and releasing the tragus against the external meatus or by increasing and decreasing the pressure in the canal with a Siegel's speculum. The subjective feeling of giddiness, nausea or vomiting with or without nystagmus indicates a positive fistula sign.

- The most common site of fistula is bony labrynth of lateral semicircular canal.

Positive fistula test: There is a fistula in the labyrinth and is still functioning. It is seen in chronic suppurative otitis media (CSOM) with cholesteatoma, tumors or trauma.

False negative fistula sign: There is a fistula in the labyrinth, but fistula test is negative. Seen in dead labyrinth or due to incorrect method of eliciting a fistula sign.

False positive fistula test: There is no fistula in the labyrinth, but fistula test is positive. This occurs in conditions:

- After stapedectomy/fenestration operations
- Congenital syphilis due to hypermobile footplate of stapes (*Hennebert's sign).*
- Endolymphatic hydrops due to any cause
- Eosinophilic granuloma.

12. Signs of Raised Intracranial Tension

13. Tests of Cerebellar Functions

14. Skull and Spine

EXAMINATION OF NOSE

1. Examination of Face and Orbit

Look for facial asymmetry, telecanthus, facial swellings, epiphora, proptosis, etc. Sensation of cheek in the infraorbital nerve area will be affected in malignancy maxilla. In the orbit, test visual acuity (Snellen's eye chart) visual field, color vision (Ishihara's chart) and pupillary reflex.

2. External Nasal Framework

Consists of skin and osteocartilaginous frame work. Look for asymmetry, deformity or swelling of nose and face.

3. Cold Spatula Test

Keep a cold metallic tongue depressor just in front of nostril. Ask the patient to breath normally with mouth closed. During expiration, look for area of condensation on the surface of tongue depressor. Fogging will be reduced on the side of nasal block.

4. Vestibule and Columella

Vestibule is the anterior skin lined area of nasal cavity. Columella separates two vestibules. This part is examined by elevating the tip of nose with examiner's fingertip. Common disorders seen here are furunculosis, redness or anterior dislocation of septum.

5. Anterior Rhinoscopy

Thudicum's speculum or St Clair Thompson's speculum are commonly used for examination. Speculum is held in left hand and nasal cavity is examined systematically. Presence/absence of nasal discharge, status of nasal mucosa, floor of nose, nasal septum and lateral wall is examined in order. Nasal mucosa is normally dull red in color. Congested mucosa is seen in inflammatory lesions.

Pale edematous mucosa is seen in allergic rhinitis. Septal deviations or spur (shelf like projection at bony-catilaginous junction of nasal septum is called spur), if present are noted. In the lateral wall, examine middle and inferior turbinates and meatus which lie lateral to the turbinates. Usually, one can see these two turbinates by anterior rhinoscopy. The meatus are noted for discharge, mass or redness. In roomy noses, superior turbinate is also seen. If nasal mass is present probing should be done. Probing is touching the mass with a probe (cotton-tipped applicator) as we palpate an abdominal mass with fingers.

Uses of Probing

To find out:

- Consistency of mass—soft in polyp, firm in turbinate hypertrophy, hard in osteoma.
- Sensitivity—inverted papilloma is usually sensitive
- Bleeding to touch—rhinosporidial mass
- Tender/not
- Shape of mass
- Number—single in antrochoanal polyp, multiple in ethmoid polyp
- Site of attachment—to know this move probe around the mass
- Cough impulse—present in mass with intracranial extension as in meningoencephalocele.

6. Palpating for Paranasal Sinus Tenderness

Remember not to elicit tenderness on both sides simultaneously.

- *Maxillary sinus* tenderness elicited by pressing on *canine fossa*. Canine fossa boundaries are: two vertical lines and two horizontal lines—upper horizontal line passing through infraorbital foramen and lower passing through superior alveolar margin. Medial vertical line passes over canine ridge and lateral through first molar teeth. Space in side these lines is canine fossa.

- *Frontal sinus* tenderness is elicited by pressing below medial end of eyebrow. Corresponds to floor of frontal sinus.
- *Ethmoid sinus* tenderness is elicited by pressing between medial canthus of eye and root of nose.

7. Posterior Rhinoscopy

Method

Patient sits facing the examiner. Explain the procedure to the patient. He is asked to open mouth and to breath quietly through nose. Depress anterior one-third of tongue with tongue depressor held in left hand. Previously warmed and temperature tested postnasal mirror is held in right hand of examiner and introduced behind soft palate without touching it. Posterior end of septum is seen as a vertical edge. Posterior choanae are seen on either side of posterior end of septum. Posterior end of turbinates are seen on lateral wall of choana. Lateral tilt of mirror will bring lateral wall of nasopharynx into view. Eustachian tube opening, elevation of eustachian cushion, and fossa of Rosenmüller noted. In children and young adults adenoid will be visible in the posterior wall and roof.

8. Examination of Nasopharynx

- *Posterior Rhinoscopy:* Explained above.
- *Digital palpation:* Not routinely done nowadays, because of use of diagnostic nasal endoscopy. Patient seated facing the examiner. Examiner stands behind the patient on his right side. Using left index finger invaginate patient's left cheek (this is to avoid accidental bite of examiner's finger by the patient). Introduce right index finger behind soft palate into nasopharynx. Palpate various parts in order. *While taking the finger out, look the tip of finger for bloodstains.*

EXAMINATION OF ORAL CAVITY AND OROPHARYNX

1. Oral Cavity

Look for mouth opening/trismus. Oral cavity is examined by retracting the cheeks by tongue depressor.

- *Lips:* Look for any fissures, clefts, angular stomatitis, etc.
- *Buccal mucosa:* Ulcer, leukoplakia, lichen planus
- *Gums and teeth:* Remove artificial teeth and dentures, if any before examination. Caries teeth, ulcers, epulis, etc. are common diseases found here.

  The arrangement of teeth and the occlusion are examined with lips open.
- *Gingivolabial and gingivobuccal sulcus:* Look for ulcer, swelling, growth, etc.
- *Anterior two-thirds of tongue:* Part of tongue anterior to circumvallate papilla and sulcus terminalis. The shape and mobility of tongue noted. In hypoglossal paresis, tongue deviates slightly to paralyzed side.
- *Hard palate*
- *Floor of mouth*—examined with tongue elevated.
- *Retromolar trigone (Coffin's Corner):* This is the triangular area behind lower third molar overlying ascending ramus of mandible and should be palpated for induration as this can be a site of hidden malignancy.

Patient is asked to lift the tip of tongue and orifices of the submandibular ducts and floor of mouth seen. The parotid duct in the cheek opposite to upper second molar tooth is inspected. Assess the orodental hygiene. Movements of soft palate are watched by asking the patient to say "Ah".

2. Oropharynx

Examined by depressing the anterior two-thirds of tongue-by-tongue depressor.

- *Anterior pillars*
- *Tonsils:* Color (red/congestion), hypertrophy, follicles, membrane, cyst, etc. are noted. Pressure by tongue depressor will squeeze the debris from tonsillar crypts in chronic tonsillitis *(Irwin Moore sign)*

  Size of the tonsil is graded as follows:
  - *Grade 1:* Medial surface of tonsil seen behind anterior pillar
  - *Grade 2:* Medial surface at the level of anterior pillar
  - *Grade 3:* Medial surface medial to the level of anterior pillar.
  - *Grade 4:* Medial surface of both tonsils touching in the midline.
- *Posterior pillars*
- *Soft palate and uvula*
- *Posterior wall of oropharynx:* Presence of postnasal drip, hypertrophied follicles, etc.
- *Posterior third of tongue (Base of tongue):* Part of tongue behind the circumvallate papillae. Best examined using indirect laryngoscopy mirror and by palpation.

Palpation

Finger palpation of base of tongue done with gloved finger and tongue kept relaxed inside oral cavity. Bidigital palpation of submandibular salivary gland and its duct done for calculus. Elongated styloid process may be felt by palpating through tonsillar fossa.

3. Indirect Laryngoscopic Examination

Patient seated facing the examiner. Procedure explained to patient. He is asked to open mouth widely and to protrude tongue. Hold tongue wrapped in gauze between thumb and middle finger.

Index finger is used to retract upper lip. Warmed and temperature tested laryngeal mirror introduced into the mouth and held firmly against soft palate and uvula. Patient is asked to breath quietly through mouth. To see movements of cords patient is asked to take deep inspiration (abduction of cords) say *Aaa* (adduction of cords) *Eee* (adduction and tension), movements of both cords are compared.

Structures seen by indirect laryngoscopy: Given along with instruments.

4. Examination of Neck

Neck nodes: Neck nodes are better palpated by standing behind the patient. Neck is minimally flexed. Nodes are palpated for size, number, consistency, tenderness and mobility.

Palpation

Palpation carried out either from front or behind. Both sides are palpated and compared. The head should be tilted forward to relax the soft tissues. Auscultation and palpation are performed for suspected vascular anomalies.

Lymph nodes are to be palpated as individual lymph node groups bimanually in sequence, recording their topographic sites, number, shape and size.

Level I : IA submental
: IB submandibular
Level II : Upper jugular
Level III : Mid jugular
Level IV : Lower jugular
Level V : Posterior triangle group
Level VI : Prelaryngeal/pretracheal/paratracheal
Level VII : Nodes of upper mediastinum

- Trachea central or not
- *Laryngeal framework:* Look for widening of laryngeal cartilage and tenderness of laryngeal framework (common in tuberculosis, perichondritis).
- *Carotid pulsations:* Feel it to know whether equal on both sides
- Jugular vein palpated for any tenderness/thickening
- *Laryngeal crepitus:* Grating sensation felt on moving laryngeal framework over prevertebral fascia.

Absent laryngeal crepitus is seen in:
- Retropharyngeal abscess
- Postcricoid malignancy
- Postirradiation carcinoma larynx
- Perichondritis of larynx
- Normal persons (17%).

System examination: Central nervous system, respiratory system, gastrointestinal and musculoskeletal systems are examined as you do in medicine.

After examination, write a summary of history and relevant positive and negative findings that help you to come to a provisional diagnosis.

CHAPTER 3

X-rays in ENT

Usually for undergraduates, in viva, radiology is limited to X-rays only.

X-RAY MASTOID

We take plain X-ray mastoids bilateral views. Commonly used views are:

- *Law's view:* Lateral oblique view of mastoid. Patients head is placed in lateral projection. The X-ray beam is directed 15° cephalocaudal. Structures (**Fig. 3.1**) seen are:
  1. Temporomandibular joint (ball and socket joint)
  2. Air of external auditory canal (Seen posterior to TM joint).

  The triangular area marked posterior to external auditory canal is the mastoid air cells. In the marked triangle;
  3. Dural plate
  4. Sinus plate
  5. Posterior wall of external auditory canal.

Q1. What are the other views for temporal bone?

Ans:

1. *Stenvers view:* This is an oblique view of skull.
2. *Towne's view:* Direction of the X-ray beam is 25–35° fronto-occipital. Both petrous pyramids can be seen in this X-ray. Usually, taken for acoustic neuroma and apical petrositis.

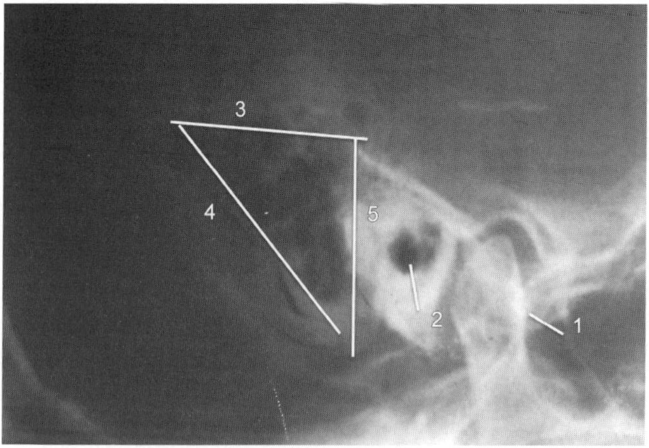

Fig. 3.1 Plain X-ray mastoid—Law's view

3. *Transorbital view:* Commonly taken to visualize internal acoustic meatus.
4. Owen's projection
5. Submentovertical view.

Q2. It is advisable to take X-ray of both side of mastoid. Why?

Ans: That is to compare the pneumatization of both sides. Pneumatization can be of three types:

1. Well-pneumatized or cellular—80%
2. *Diploetic:* Contains both marrow spaces and air cells—10%
3. *Sclerotic or acellular:* This can be as developmental or after repeated infection—10%.

Q3. What are the uses of taking X-ray mastoid?

Ans:

1. To know the type of pneumatization (**Figs 3.2 to 3.4**).
2. To know the anatomical landmarks; as:
   a. *Sinus plate:* Which can be normal/anteriorly positioned
   b. *Dural plate:* Sometimes low lying, so that there is danger of injury during mastoid exploration.

3. To know presence of bone erosion **(Fig. 3.7)**:
   a. *Cholesteatoma*—smooth cavity with surrounding sclerosis.
   b. *Postsurgical (after mastoid exploration)*—smooth cavity
   c. Diseases affecting mastoid and middle ear as in malignancy.
4. To find out masked mastoiditis—clouding of mastoid air cells with dissolution of intercellular septum **(Figs 3.5 and 3.6)**.

Q4. What is Körner's septum?

Ans: It is petrosquamous suture persisting as bony plate, called *petrosquamous lamina*. Körner's septum is surgically important as it may cause difficulty in locating the mastoid antrum which may lie deep to it. Thus, it can lead to incomplete removal of disease in mastoidectomy.

SOME X-RAYS OF MASTOID LATERAL OBLIQUE VIEW (LAW'S VIEW)

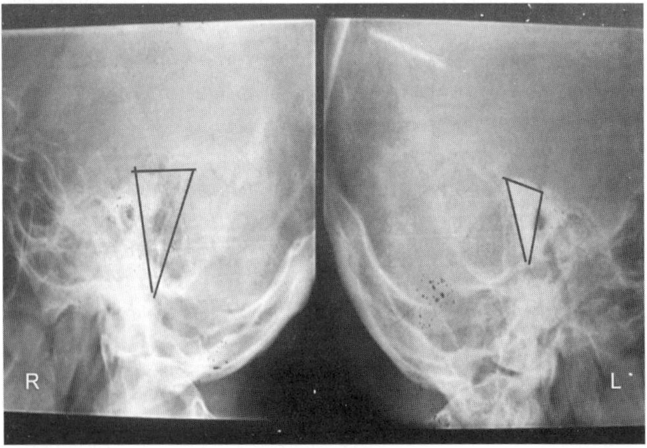

Fig. 3.2 Diploic mastoid air cells on right side and sclerotic on left side

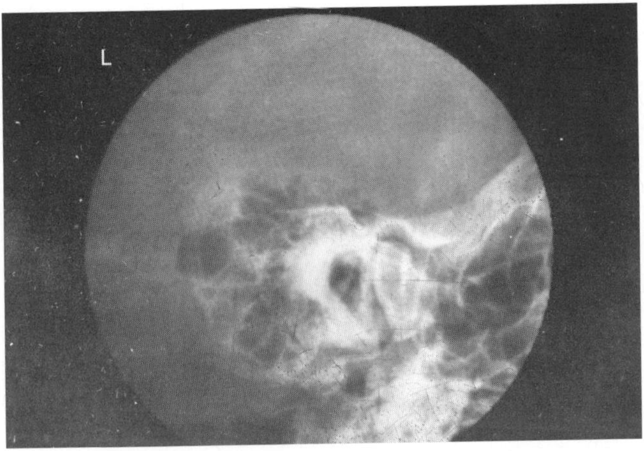

Fig. 3.3 Plain X-ray mastoid lateral oblique view showing cellular mastoid

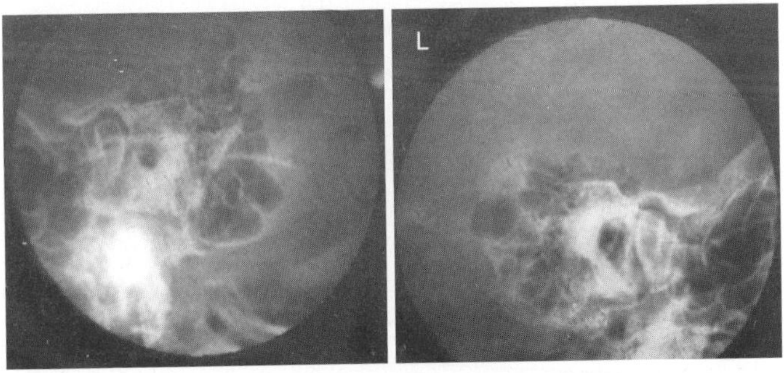

Fig. 3.4 Plain X-ray mastoid both sides showing cellular mastoid

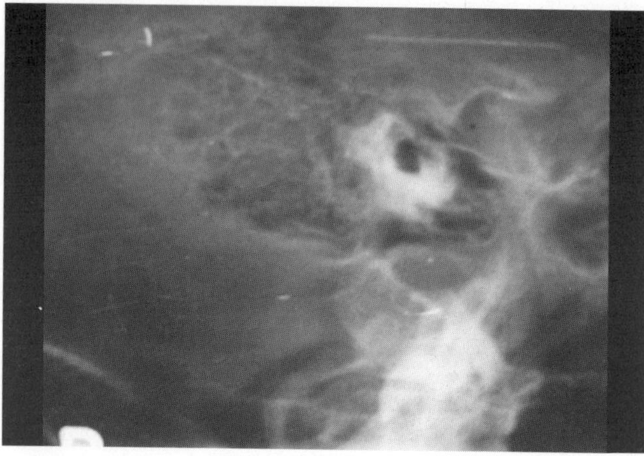

Fig. 3.5 X-ray of mastoiditis showing clouding of air cells and dissolution of intercellular septum

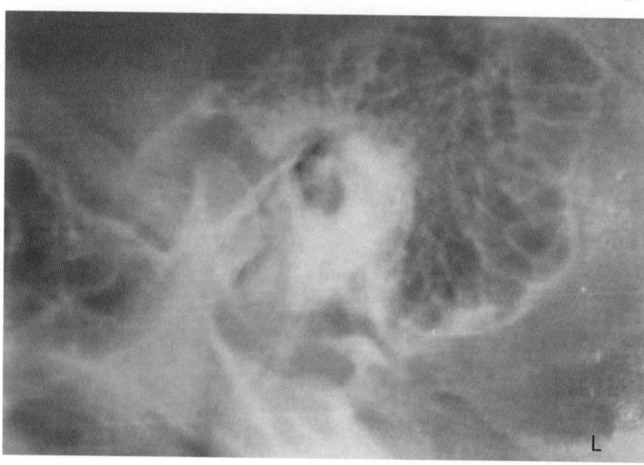

Fig. 3.6 X-ray of mastoid lateral oblique view left side showing clouding of air cells and dissolution of intercellular septum. Probable diagnosis is acute mastoiditis leftside

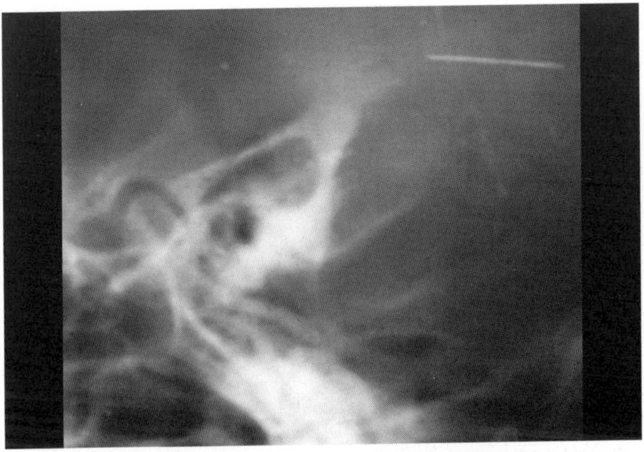

Fig. 3.7 Plain X-ray mastoid lateral oblique view showing cavity inside mastoid

NOSE AND PARANASAL SINUSES

Nose

In nose, X-ray is taken for nasal bone fracture. Plain X-ray (lateral view) of nasal bone (both right and left lateral views) are taken. Fracture line and depression or elevation of fractured segment is seen in X-ray **(Figs 3.8A and B)**. *Groove for ethmoid nerve and vessels run downwards and forward and it should not be mistaken for fracture line.*

Q1. The most common fracture of faciomaxillary skeleton is
Ans: Fracture nasal bone (40% of facial fractures).

Q2. The most common cause of fracture nasal bone is
Ans: Trauma.

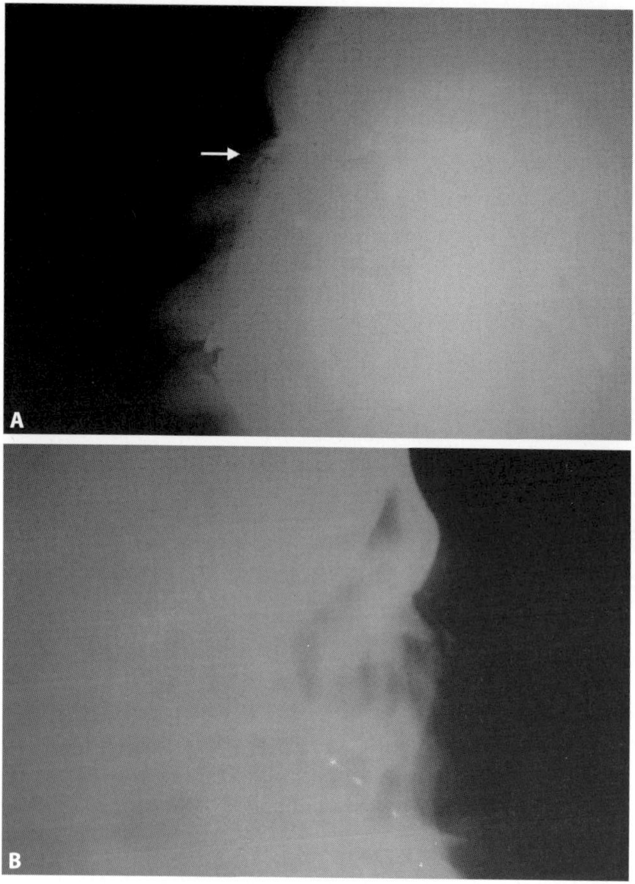

Figs 3.8A and B X-ray nasal bone lateral view showing fracture of nasal bone

Q3. What are the types of nasal bone fracture?

Ans:

1. *Depressed:* Due to frontal blow. A severe frontal blow will cause an *open book fracture*
2. *Angulated:* Due to lateral blow.

Q4. What are the types of fracture nasal septum?

Ans: Two types:

1. *Chevallet fracture:* Fracture line runs *vertically* from anterior nasal spine upwards to dorsum of nose
2. *Jarjavay's fracture: Horizontal* fracture line from just above anterior nasal spine, going backwards to vomer.

Q5. How will you diagnose nasal bone fracture?

Ans: Nasal bone fracture is diagnosed clinically:

a. History of trauma face and pain root/dorsum nose. Associated complaints such as epistaxis, nasal deformity, nasal block, etc. will be present.
b. Tenderness and crepitus at root of nose. Nasal deformity may or may not be there.
c. X-ray nasal bone lateral view is only for documentation purpose.

Q6. How will you treat fracture nasal bone?

Ans:

- Simple fracture without displacement need conservative treatment only.
- Fracture with displacement needs reduction. Presence of edema interferes with accurate reduction. So, if patient comes to you immediately after sustaining injury, before appearance of edema, it can be reduced by closed method
- Walsham's forceps for nasal bone and Asch's forceps for nasal septal fractures.
- Depressed fractures can also be reduced by BP handle (handle of Bard Parker knife) guided by digital pressure.

- If edema has developed, wait for 7–10 days for subsidence of edema and do closed reduction.
- If patient comes after 3–6 weeks with malunited fracture treatment is rhinoplasty.

Q7. What is Le-Fort fracture?

Ans: They are fracture of maxilla:

Three types:

Le-Fort I—Transverse (Guerin) fracture result in floating palate

Le-Fort II—Pyramidal fracture

Le-Fort III—Craniofacial disjunction.

Q8. What are Tripod fracture?

Ans: Fracture zygoma.

Paranasal Sinus

Q1. What are the X-ray views for paranasal sinuses (PNS)?

Ans:

1. *30° occipitomental view (Water's view)* ***(Fig. 3.9)****:* This is the most common view taken for sinuses. X-ray is taken in nose-chin position. In this view, all sinuses including nasal cavity and septum is visualized. Water's view with open mouth (Modified water's view) shows sphenoid sinus also. This view is ideal for maxillary sinus.
2. *Occipitofrontal view (Caldwell view):* This is ideal view for frontal sinus. It also shows ethmoid sinus, nasal cavity and orbit.
3. *Submentovertical view (skull base):* This view is useful for demonstrating sphenoid sinus. It also shows nasopharynx, petrous apex, posterior wall of maxillary sinus and fracture of zygomatic arch.
4. *Lateral oblique view for ethmoids:* In plain X-ray, *normal sinus appear as air-filled translucent cavities.* Opacity can be caused by fluid, thickened mucosa or tumors.

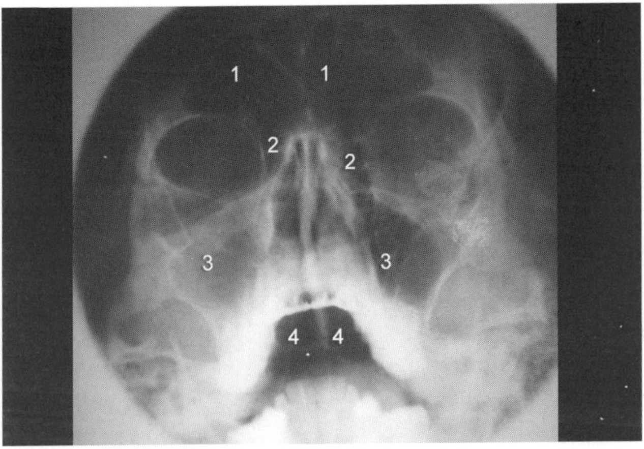

Fig. 3.9 Plain X-ray (Paranasal sinus) Water's view with open mouth showing sinuses: 1. Frontal sinus; 2. Ethmoid sinus; 3. Maxillary sinus; 4. Sphenoid sinus. We compare haziness of sinuses with that of orbital cavity. Here there is haziness of right maxillary sinus

X-ray appearance of normal frontal sinus is called *Scalloping* (meaning: outer shell) appearance. The absence of scalloping with expansion of sinus cavity is seen in frontal mucocele.

Water's view in standing position may show air-fluid level in maxillary sinus, in case of acute sinusitis **(Fig. 3.10)**.

Q2. Differential diagnosis of opacity maxillary sinus (Figs 3.11 to 3.13).

Ans: Mucocele, pyocele, sinusitis, dental cyst, dentigerous cyst, hemosinus, retention cyst, mucosal thickening, antral polyp, benign or malignant lesions of maxilla.

Q3. Name conditions causing calcification in X-ray (PNS).

Ans: Inverted papilloma, meningioma, chordoma and chondrosarcoma.

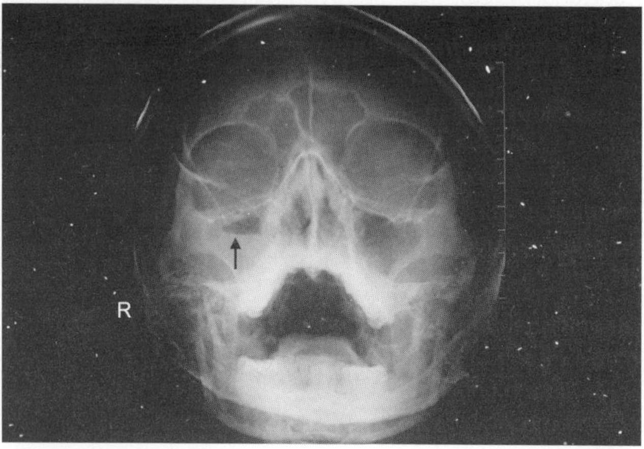

Fig. 3.10 Plain X-ray (Paranasal sinuses) (Water's view) showing air-fluid level in right maxillary sinus. Suggestive of right acute maxillary sinusitis

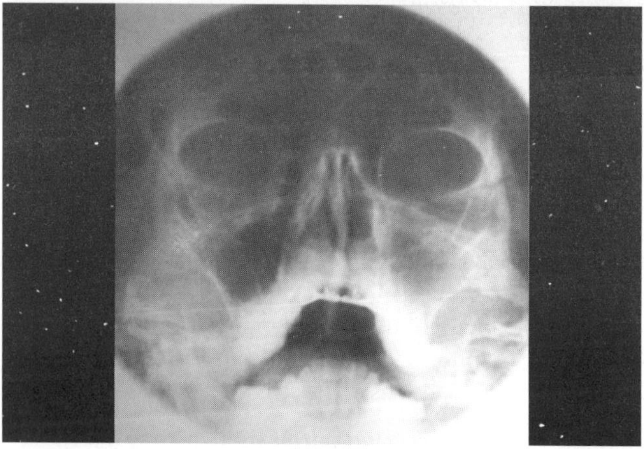

Fig. 3.11 Plain X-ray (paranasal sinus) Water's view with open mouth, showing opacity in left maxillary sinus

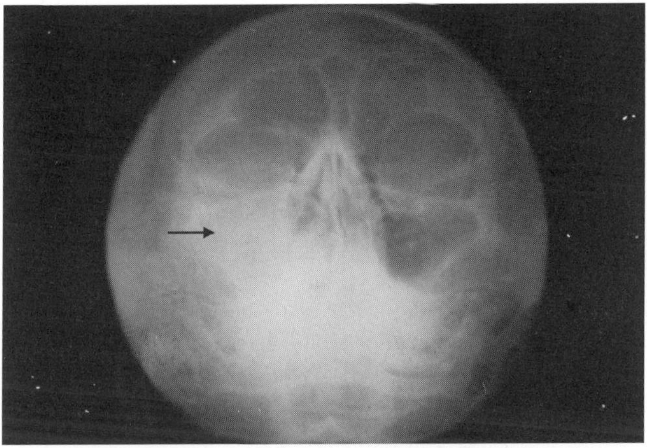

Fig. 3.12 Plain X-ray (Paranasal sinuses) Water's view showing haziness right maxillary sinus

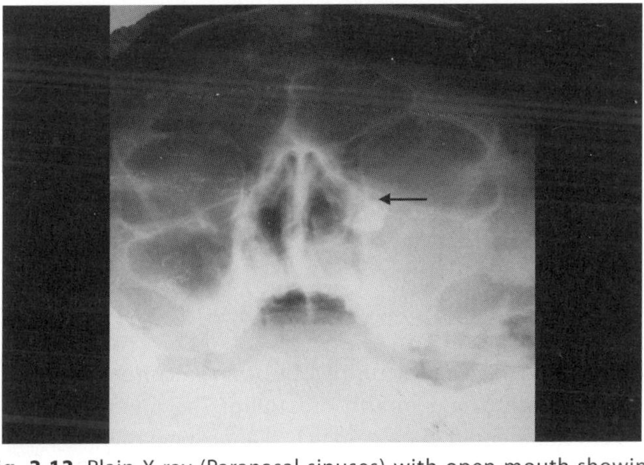

Fig. 3.13 Plain X-ray (Paranasal sinuses) with open mouth showing opacity in left maxillary sinus with a radiopaque area medial wall of left maxillary sinus. Diagnosis is dentigerous cyst left maxillary sinus (*dentigerous cyst arises from follicle around an unerupted tooth*)

Q4. List the complications of chronic sinusitis.

Ans:

A. *Local:*
1. Mucocele/pyocele
2. Mucous retention cyst
3. Osteomylitis (most common is of frontal bone)

B. *Orbital:*
1. Preseptal cellulitis
2. Subperiosteal abscess
3. Orbital cellulitis
4. Orbital abscess
5. Superior orbital fissure syndrome
6. Orbital apex syndrome

C. *Intracranial:*
1. Meningitis
2. Extradural abscess
3. Subdural abscess
4. Brain abscess
5. Cavernous sinus thrombosis

Q5. What is the treatment of choice for chronic sinusitis?

Ans: Functional endoscopic sinus surgery (FESS).

Q6. If no facilities for doing FESS, what is the surgical option for chronic maxillary sinusitis?

Ans: Caldwell-Luc operation.

NASOPHARYNX

- X-ray nasopharynx lateral view **(Fig. 3.14)** is used to grade adenoid hypertrophy.
- Child with this X-ray picture will be having recurrent rhinorrhea with snoring and mouth-breathing. The investigation to confirm adenoid hypertrophy is diagnostic nasal endoscopy and CT Scan nose and nasopharynx.
- Adenoid is poorly developed at birth and is radiologically visible in all infants by 4–6 months.

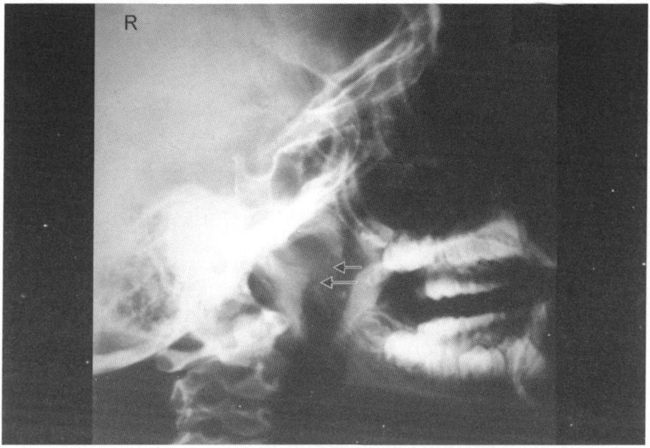

Fig. 3.14 X-ray nasopharynx lateral view showing adenoid hypertrophy (arrows)

- Antrochoanal polyp may also show a soft tissue density, but a column of air is seen between the mass and posterior wall of nasopharynx. This column of air differentiate AC polyp from other nasopharyngeal mass arising from posterior wall of nasopharynx like adenoid, angiofibroma, etc.
- In nasopharyngeal angiofibroma, lateral X-ray skull shows anterior bowing of posterior wall of maxilla due to tumor enlarging in the pterygopalatine fossa. This is known as an *Antral sign* or *Holman Miller sign.*
- Adenoid have a feel like *bag of worms* on palpation.
- *Adenoid facies*: Child presents with dull look, pinched nostril, open mouth, hitched up upper lip, protruding upper incisors and high-arched palate.

X-RAY NECK

Soft Tissue Neck Lateral View (Fig. 3.15)

This view helps in the diagnosis of:

- Foreign bodies of larynx/pharynx—presence and location **(Figs 3.16 and 3.17)**
- Acute epiglottitis—epiglottis edematous and shows *Thumb sign*
- Retropharyngeal abscess—there will be widening of prevertebral soft-tissue shadow. *To call as abscess, Widening should be more than 3/4th diameter of corresponding cervical vertebral body.*
    - *Acute retropharyngeal abscess* ***(Figs 3.18 and 3.19):*** It is most common cause of this in adult is penetrating injury mainly due to foreign body. In children, most common cause of acute retropharyngeal abscess is retropharyngeal lymphadenitis (*Glands of Henle*)
    - *Chronic retropharyngeal abscess* is caused by tuberculosis of cervical spine (Pott's spine). X-ray evidence of destruction and collapse of intervertebral disc will be present **(Fig. 3.19)**.

Q1. Which is the most common site of foreign body (FB) upper digestive tract?

Ans: Cricopharynx.

Q2. What is the treatment of foreign body hypopharynx?

Ans: Whether FB pharynx/esophagus treatment is hypopharyngoscopy/esophagoscopy and FB removal using FB removal forceps under local or general anesthesia.

Q3. A case of acute retropharyngeal abscess develops fever, dyspnea and chest pain. What is the probable diagnosis?

Ans: Acute mediastinitis (Space of Gillette freely communicates with the superior mediastinum).

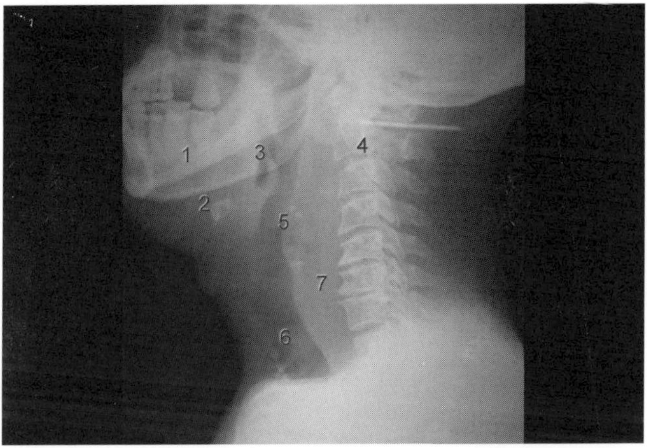

Fig. 3.15 Plain X-ray soft tissue neck lateral view showing acute retropharyngeal abscess: 1. Lower border of mandible; 2. Hyoid bone; 3. Epiglottis; 4. Cervical vertebra; 5. Laryngeal cartilages (calcified); 6. Tracheal aircolumn, 7; Prevertebral soft tissues (Retropharyngeal space)

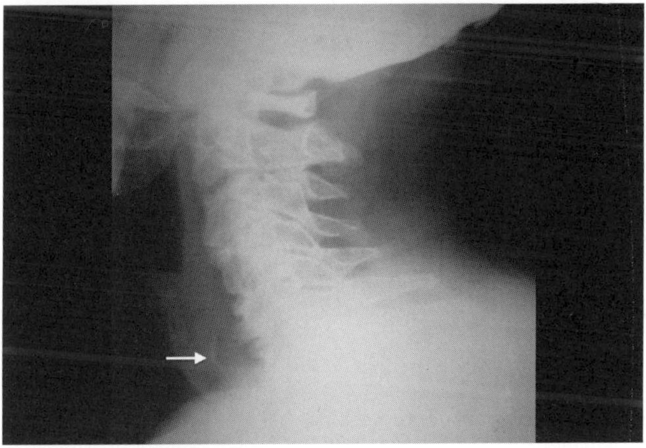

Fig. 3.16 X-ray soft tissue neck (lateral view) showing radiodense linear opacity opposite to C5–C6 vertebrae. *Diagnosis:* Foreign body in hypopharynx, probably fish bone

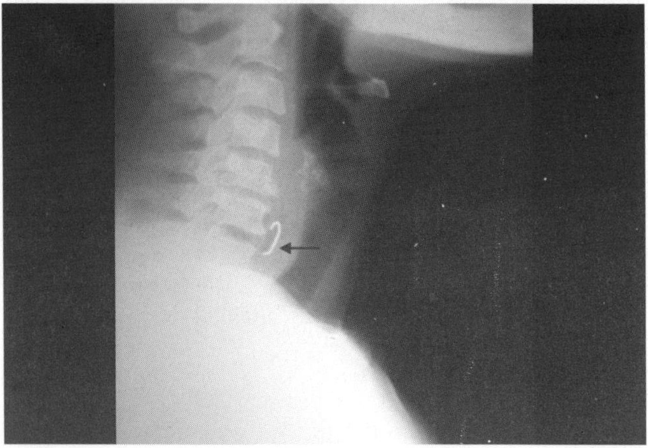

Fig. 3.17 X-ray soft tissue neck (lateral view) showing radiodense opacity opposite to C6–C7 vertebrae. *Diagnosis:* Foreign body hypopharynx (stapler pin)

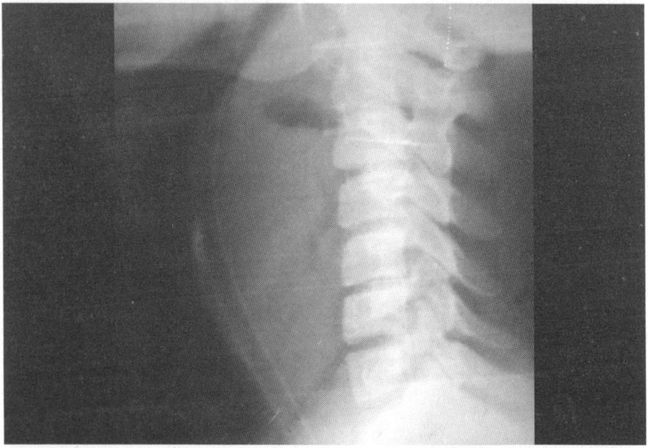

Fig. 3.18 X-ray soft tissue neck (lateral view) showing widening of retropharyngeal space starting from the level of hyoid bone with air-fluid level. Straightening of cervical vertebra present. Compression of tracheal air column and presence of shadow of nasogastric tube. *Diagnosis:* Acute retropharyngeal abscess

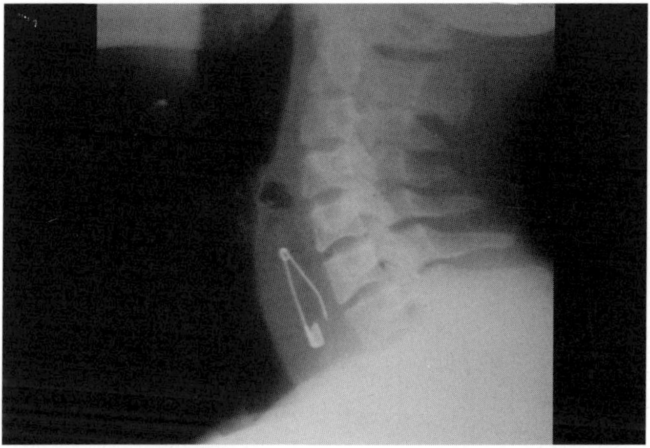

Fig. 3.19 X-ray soft tissue neck (lateral view) showing shadow of open safety pin in the retropharyngeal space opposite to C5–C7. Since the pointed end is downwards, it is relatively safe. Removed with special forceps called Clerf-Arrowsmith safety pin-closing forceps

Q4. What is Lemierre's syndrome?

Ans: Internal jugular vein thrombophlebitis secondary to deep neck space infections involving carotid space.

Q5. How will you treat chronic retropharyngeal abscess?

Ans: Start on full course of antitubercular therapy (ATT). Abscess is drained externally through a vertical incision along the sternomastoid muscle.

Q6. Why in cricopharynx (Fig. 3.20)?

Ans: Shadow is seen in coronal plane. Opening of cricopharynx is located in coronal plane.

Q7. How can you confirm that it is in cricopharynx?

Ans: Confirmed by taking X-ray soft tissue neck lateral view **(Fig. 3.21)**.

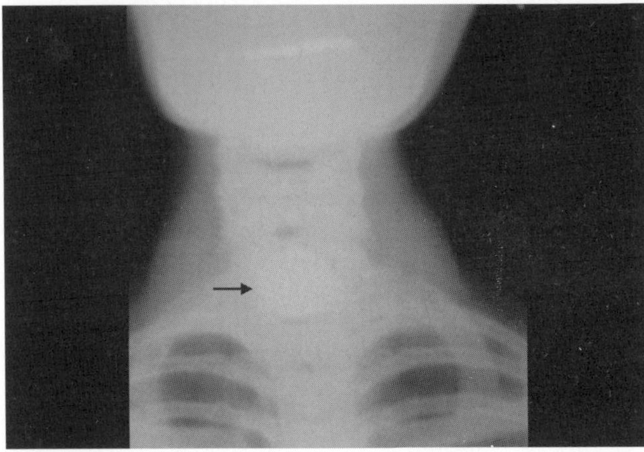

Fig. 3.20 X-ray neck with upper chest anteroposterior view showing a radiopaque round shadow (probably a coin) in cricopharynx

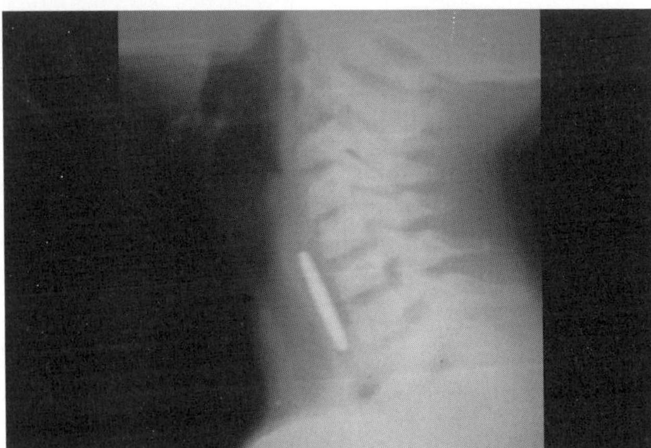

Fig. 3.21 X-ray soft tissue neck (lateral view) showing shadow of radiopaque foreign body opposite to C5–C7 vertebrae

Q8. What is the treatment of acute retropharyngeal abscess?

Ans: Retropharyngeal abscess is a serious emergency:

- Admit the patient
- Start on intravenous broad-spectrum antibiotic
- Correct fluid and electrolyte imbalance, if any
- Under local/general anesthesia, do hypopharyngoscopy/esophagoscopy and remove FB, if any, using FB removal forceps. Using endoscopic scissors put a *cruciate incision* over most bulging point of the abscess and drain pus using suction.
- If there is *chance of airway compromise, do a tracheostomy* prior to endoscopy.

CHAPTER 4

Instruments in ENT

The instruments commonly asked in viva and objective structured clinical examination (OSCE) only are discussed here.

INSTRUMENTS IN EAR

Simpson's Aural Syringe (Fig. 4.1)

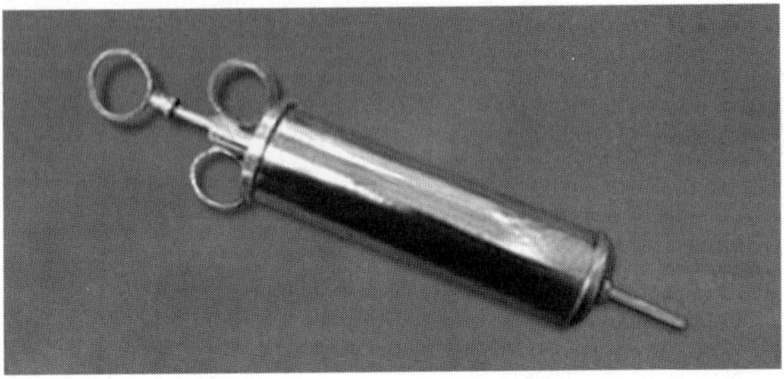

Fig. 4.1 Simpson's aural syringe

Q1. What are the uses?

Ans:

- Removal of foreign body ear
- Removal of wax ear.

Q2. What are the contraindications?

Ans:

- Perforated tympanic membrane as in acute suppurative otitis media (ASOM)/chronic suppurative otitis media (CSOM)

- Hygroscopic foreign body (FB) (Vegetable FB like peanut)
- Cerebrospinal fluid (CSF) otorrhea
- Otitis externa.

Q3. What are the complications of aural syringing?

Ans:

- Canal trauma
- Tympanic membrane rupture
- Activation of latent otitis media
- Vasovagal attack
- Vertigo due to stimulation of labyrinth.

Q4. What are the precautions to be taken while syringing?

Ans:

- Water should be at body temperature (37°) to prevent stimulation of labyrinth
- Direction of water should be towards posterosuperior canal wall in order to protect tympanic membrane from force of water and also to push the FB from behind
- Tip of syringe should be blunt
- *Always do dry mopping after syringing,* so as to prevent superadded fungal infections of the canal.

Q5. How will you syringe an ear?

Ans: Patient seated in front of examiner. Kidney tray is kept below the ear and sheet put around the shoulder of the patient to avoid soiling with water. Fill the syringe with saline at body temperature and push with tip directed towards posterosuperior canal wall.

Q6. What are the causes of impaction of FB?

Ans:

- Curvature of external auditory canal (EAC) is S shaped
- Presence of Anterior tympanic recess in the canal
- Edema EAC due to instrumentation/release of toxins from FB.

Q7. Which is the narrowest part of EAC?

Ans: It is the isthmus which lies 5 mm away from tympanic membrane.

Q8. What is the capacity of syringe?

Ans: 150 mL in adult.

Hartmann's Ear Forceps (Fig. 4.2)

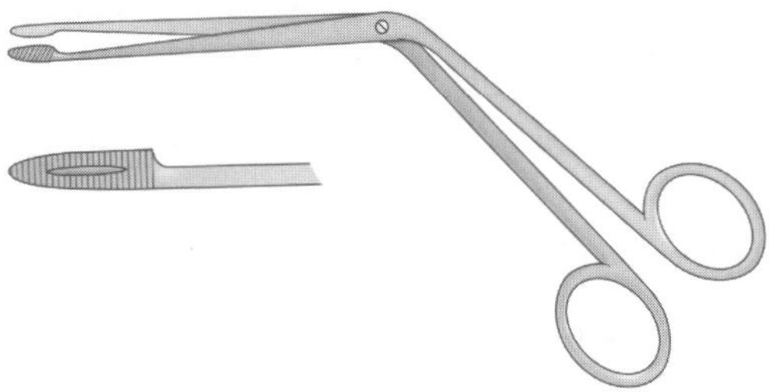

Fig. 4.2 Hartmann's ear forceps
Note the serrations inside the tip to increase the grip

Uses

1. For ear-packing
2. Removal of FB from ear.

Mollison's Self-retaining Hemostatic Mastoid Retractor (Fig. 4.3)

Q1. Enumerate the uses of this.

Ans:

- Used in surgeries to harvest temporalis fascia
- In all mastoid surgeries
- Laryngofissure surgery
- Tracheostomy

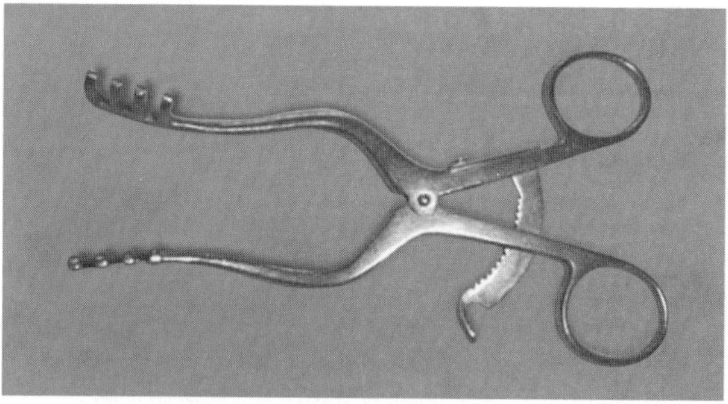

Fig. 4.3 Mollison's self-retaining mastoid retractor

- External ethmoidectomy (Lynch Howarth's)
- Frontal trephining.

Q2. What are the advantages of this instrument?

Ans:

- As it is self-retaining, no assistance is needed to hold this instrument
- Secure hemostasis by lateral pressure over the tissues.
- It retracts the tissues away from the field of surgery.

Jobson Horne's Probe and Ring Curette (Fig. 4.4)

Q1. What are the uses?

Ans: With the curette end we can remove wax, foreign body, granulation tissue, etc. Probe end is used as cotton swab carrier to clean external auditory canal and also to probe nasal masses.

Siegle's Pneumatic Speculum (Fig. 4.5)

Q1. What are the uses?

Ans:

- To get a magnified view (X 2.5) of tympanic membrane
- To assess the mobility of TM

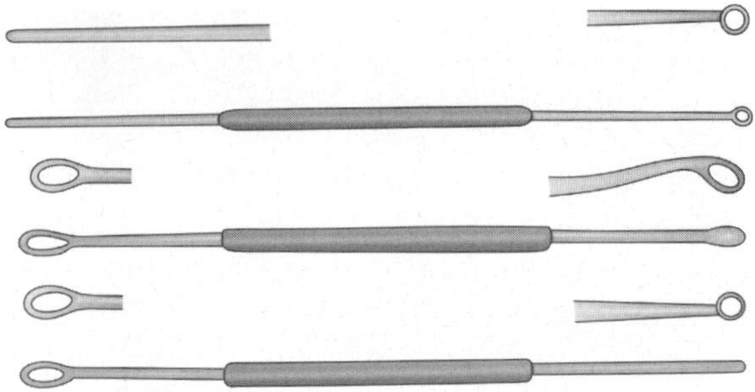

Fig. 4.4 Jobson Horne's probe of different sizes

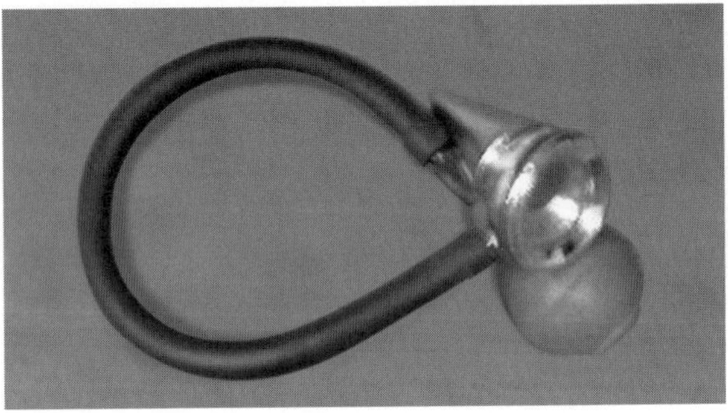

Fig. 4.5 Siegle's pneumatic speculum

- To increase and decrease the pressure of external canal in doing fistula test.
- To elicit Browne's sign in glomus tumor and in Gelle's test
- To differentiate perforation from retraction pocket.

Gardiner Brown Tuning Fork (Fig. 4.6)

Q1. Name the parts of tuning fork.

Ans: Prongs, free end, shoulder, base, stem and foot piece.

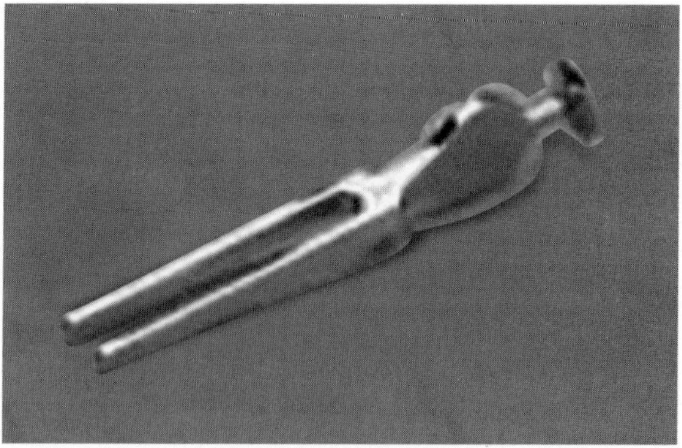

Fig. 4.6 Tuning fork

Q2. Which frequency is used commonly? Why?
Ans: Given along with ENT examination (Chapter 2).

Q3. What are the uses of tuning fork?
Ans: Used to assess the type and degree of hearing loss.

Different types of tuning fork test and methods to do, so is already discussed in examination of ear.

Jenkin's Mastoid Gouge (Figs 4.7A and B)

Used in Caldwell-Luc operation, submucous resection (SMR), mastoid surgery, etc. Nowadays, its use is limited because of high speed drill.

Gouge: Single bevel, edge is curved
Chisel: Single bevel
Osteotome: Double bevel.

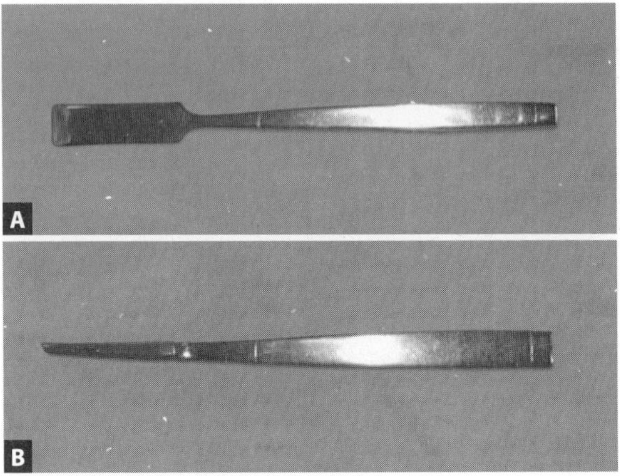

Figs 4.7A and B Jenkin's mastoid gouge. Note the edge

INSTRUMENTS FOR NOSE

Thudicum's Nasal Speculum (Figs 4.8 to 4.10)

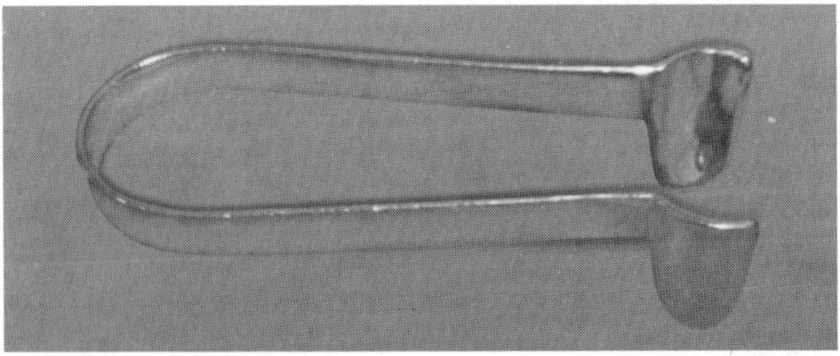

Fig. 4.8 Thudicum's nasal speculum

Pilcher's Nasal Speculum (Fig. 4.9)

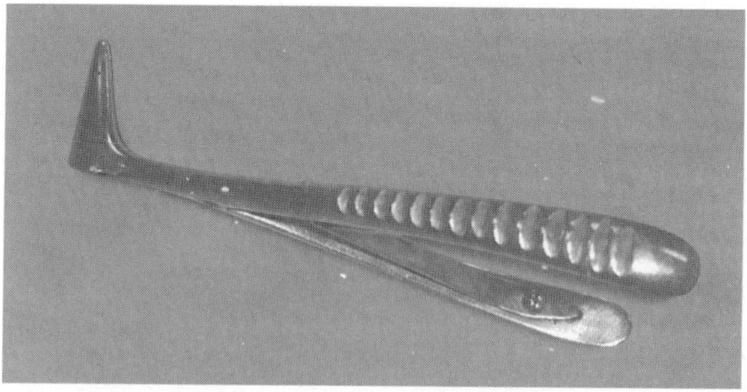

Fig. 4.9 Pilcher's nasal speculum

Q1. What are the uses?

Ans: To do anterior rhinoscopy, septal surgeries, anterior nasal packing, removal of foreign body nose, antral wash out.

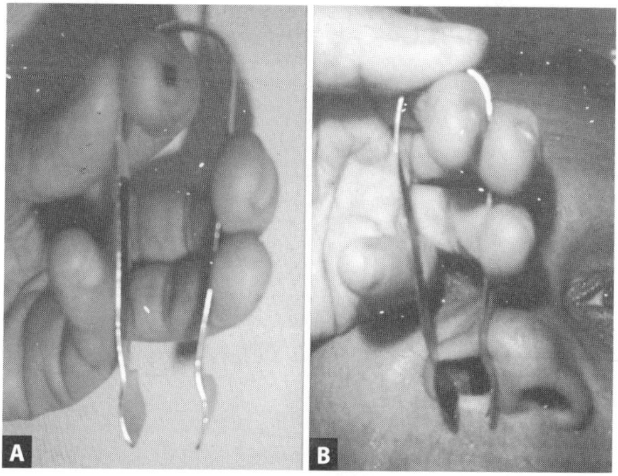

Figs 4.10A and B Thudicum's speculum held in left hand. Close blades before introduction and removal

St Clair Thompson's Long-bladed Nasal Speculum (Fig. 4.11)

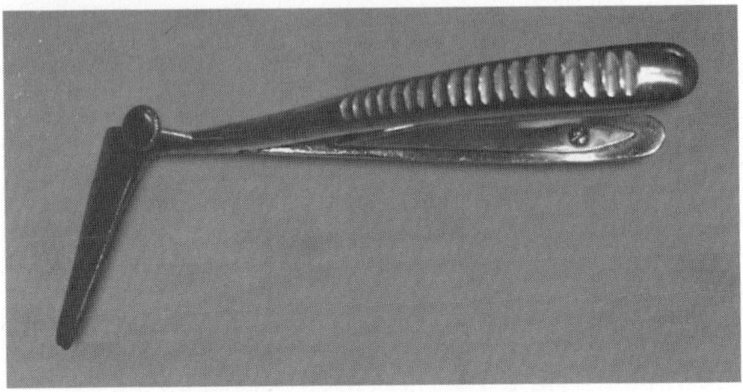

Fig. 4.11 St Clair Thompson's nasal speculum

This is used only after anesthetizing the nose as it can cause pain and discomfort to the patient. Used in surgeries of nose like septoplasty, SMR, polypectomy, etc.

Rose Eustachian Tube Catheter (Fig. 4.12)

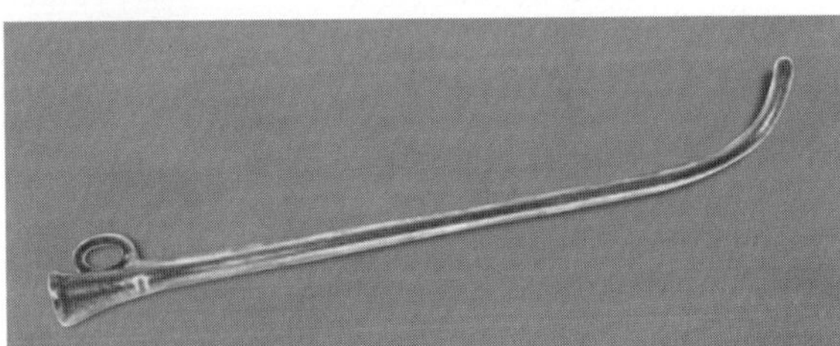

Fig. 4.12 Eustachian tube catheter. It is 12–15 cm long metallic catheter

Q1. What are the uses?

Ans:

- Removal foreign body nose
- To know the patency of Eustachian tube (not done nowadays)
- Used as suction cannula.

Q2. Name tests of eustachian dysfunction?

Ans:

- Valsalva's maneuver
- Toynbee's maneuver
- Frenzel maneuver
- Politzerization
- Siegalization
- ET cannulation
- Radiopaque dye injected and X-ray
- Nasal endoscopy
- ET endoscopy
- Sonotubometry
- Impedence audiometry
- CT scan
- 3D CT scan
- MRI scan.

Q3. How will you do Valsalva maneuver?

Ans: Ask the patient to blow out with mouth and nostril closed and note the outward movement of tympanic membrane.

Q4. How will you do Toynbee maneuver?

Ans: Ask the patient to swallow after closing nostril and mouth. TM will move inwards.

Q5. How will you do Frenzel's maneuver?

Ans: Ask the patient to move the tongue up against the palate after closing nose and mouth. TM will move inwards. This is the ideal method to test ET function among the three.

Tilley Lichtwitz Antrum Puncture Trocar and Cannula (Fig. 4.13)

Q1. What are the uses?

Ans:

- To drain pus from maxillary sinus in case of chronic maxillary sinusitis

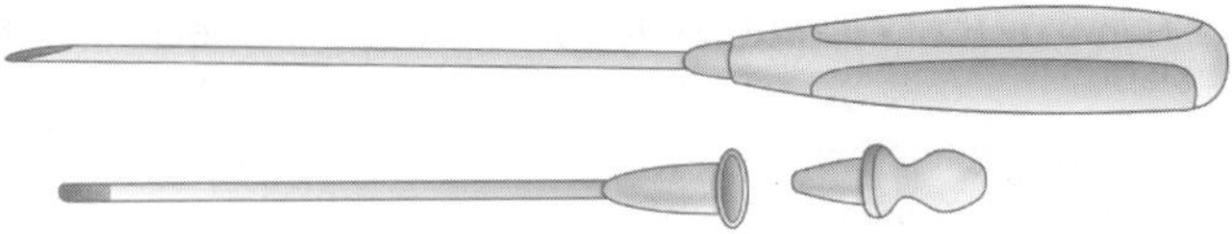

Fig. 4.13 Tilley Lichtwitz trocar and cannula

- Proof puncture in case of malignancy maxilla (this is to diagnose early malignancy by aspirating the fluid inside the sinus for malignant cells).

Q2. Name the contraindications of antral wash.

Ans:

- Acute sinusitis/rhinitis: Age below 3 years
- Bleeding disorders
- Clotting disorders.

Q3. What are the complications?

Ans:

- Puncture of orbital wall resulting in orbital injury or cellulitis (during washing ask to keep the eyes open and note any swelling/emphysema.
- Air embolism
- Bleeding
- Puncture of soft tissues resulting in swelling cheek.

Q4. How will you do antral wash?

Procedure: Patient position is semi-sitting/supine. Anesthetize inferior meatus with 4% xylocaine-dipped cotton pledgets. Hold the trocar and cannula in right hand in pen-holding fashion. Position it 1.5 cm behind the anterior end of inferior turbinate. Direction of trocar is kept towards the ipsilateral ear tragus. By screwing motion of hand, puncture the bone. A give away feel is got on puncturing the medial wall of maxillary sinus. The trocar is withdrawn and cannula-placed properly in the sinus cavity. Irrigate sinus cavity with normal saline at body temperature.

Water flows out through mouth and nose and collected in the kidney tray placed below chin.

- If sinus ostium is blocked washed out fluid will not come out of nose. In that case a second opening is made along the side of the first one.
- *Watson William's* trocar and cannula is used for sphenoid sinus washing.

Higginson's Rubber Syringe (Fig. 4.14)

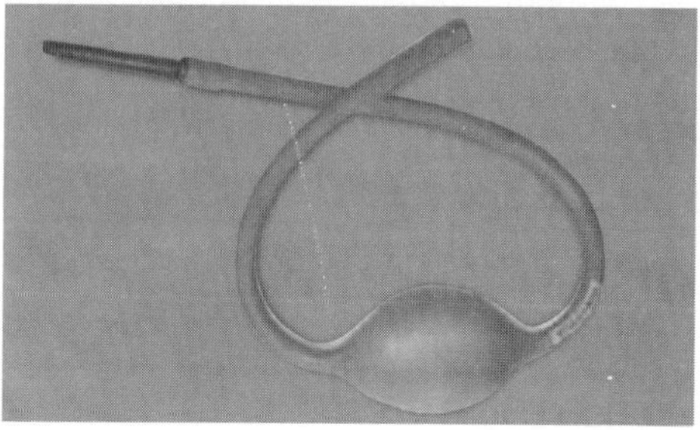

Fig. 4.14 Higginson's rubber syringe

Q1. What are the uses?

Ans: For saline nasal douche, as postoperative care after FESS, atrophic rhinitis and for antral washing after antral puncture

- Made of red rubber
- Capacity is 50 mL
- *Parts:* Bulb, rubber tubing with valve end and nozzle end
- There are *two valves* inside syringe; one at valve end and another inside the bulb.

Ballenger's Swivel Knife (Fig. 4.15) (Swivel = Swing/Like a Giant Wheel)

It is used in submucous resection (SMR) of septum. Cutting blade rotates around two bars for 360 degrees. So during surgery, it can

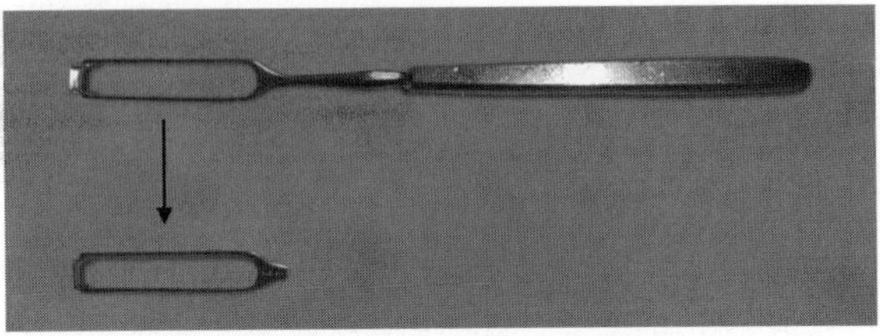

Fig. 4.15 Ballenger's swivel knife

be positioned without rotating the instrument and entire septal cartilage except caudal and dorsal strut can be removed without taking the knife outside.

Walsham Forceps and Asch's Forceps

Used to refracture and realign fracture nasal bone and displaced septum.

Walsham Forceps (**Fig. 4.16**)

Separate forceps for right and left side.

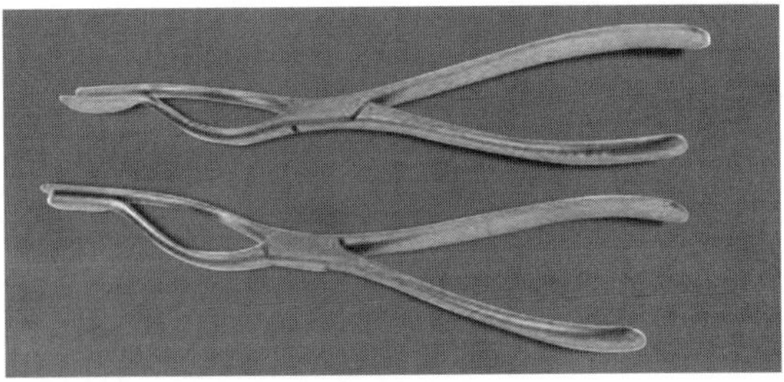

Fig. 4.16 Walsham forceps

This is used to refracture and disimpact the fractured nasal bones, and then they are realigned.

Asch's Forceps ***(Figs 4.17A and B)***

The Asch's forceps is used to elevate and straighten the septum.

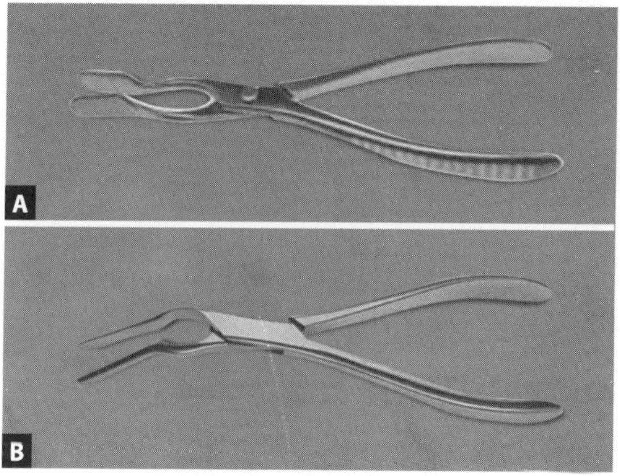

Figs 4.17A and B Asch's forceps

Tilley's Nasal Dressing Forceps (Fig. 4.18)

Used for anterior nasal packing.

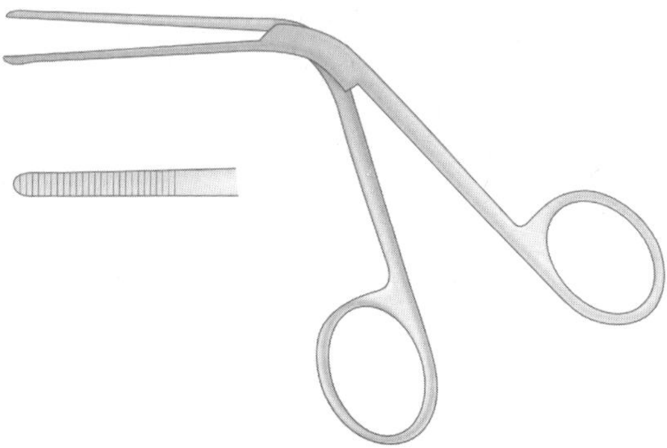

Fig. 4.18 Tilley's nasal dressing forceps

St Clair Thompson Quincy Draining Forceps (Fig. 4.19)

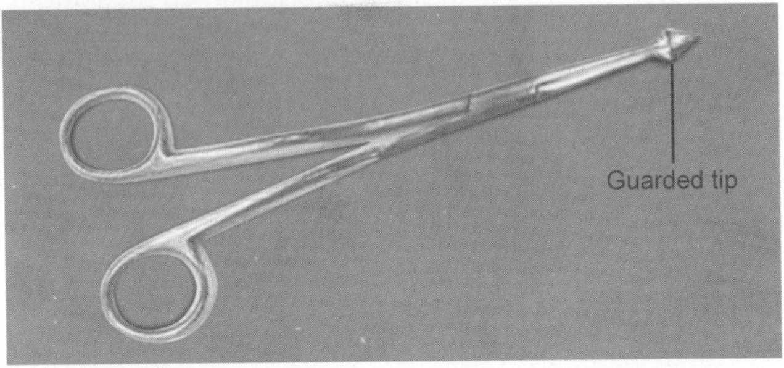

Fig. 4.19 St Clair Thompson quincy draining forceps

Uses: For draining pus in peritonsillar abscess (Quincy).

Advantage: Tip of forceps is guarded.

Sites of drainage:

- Most prominent part of swelling
- Just lateral to the intersection of an imaginary line drawn from the base of uvula with another imaginary line drawn along anterior faucial pillar
  - Always do aspiration with wide bore needle before doing I and D, because aneurysm of ICA or vascular tumor of parapharyngeal space can mimic quincy
  - Put cruciate incision with forceps.

Q4. What will happen, if you do not drain a quincy?

Ans:

- Abscess may rupture spontaneously and cause aspiration and asphyxia
- Spread of infection to other neck spaces forming parapharyngeal/retropharyngeal abscess or superior mediastinitis

- Systemic sprad of infection causing septicemia and multiple abscess
- Chance of laryngeal edema and stridor.

Q5. How quincy causes superior mediastinal abscess?
Ans: Infection spread through carotid sheet which is valveless and direct access to superior mediastinum (Lincoln's highway)

INSTRUMENTS FOR ADENOTONSILLECTOMY

Boyle Davis Mouth Gag and Doughty's Tongue Blade (Figs 4.20 and 4.21)

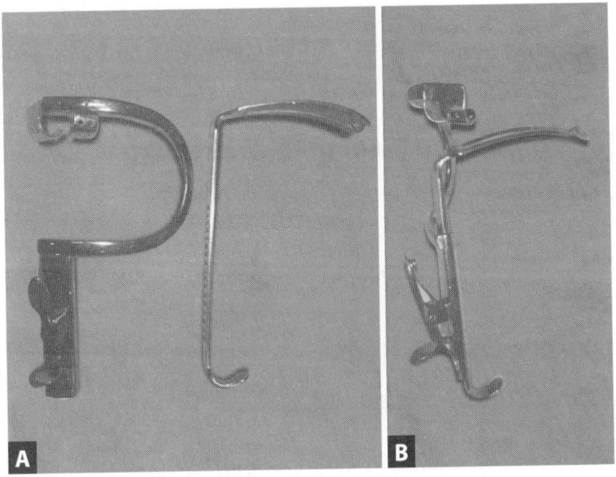

Figs 4.20A and B Boyle Davis mouth gag and Doughty's tongue blade

Uses: To open oral cavity in surgeries like tonsillectomy, adenoidectomy, operations of palate (Wilson's), nasopharynx.

Q1. What are the parts?
Ans: 1. Tongue plate 2. Jaw piece.

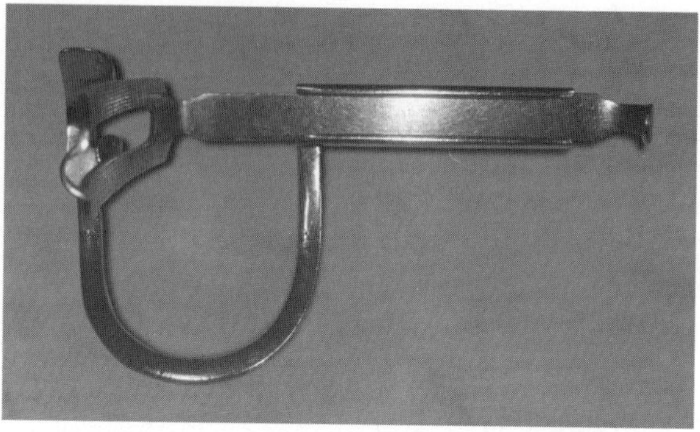

Fig. 4.21 Mouth gag and tongue blade—assembled

Q2. Name two other types of mouth gag?
Ans: Dingman and Doyen Jansen.

Draffin's Bipod and Magauran's Plate (Figs 4.22A and B)

Magauran's plate is for holding Draffin's bipod.

St Clair Thomson Adenoid Curette with/without Guard (Fig. 4.23)

Used in adenoidectomy.

Q1. What are the uses of guard?
Ans:

- Ensures complete removal of adenoid tissue
- Prevents slipping of adenoid tissue into larynx and later aspiration pneumonia.

Denis Brown Tonsil Holding Forceps (Figs 4.24A and B)

Used to hold the tonsil during dissection. Appearance is similar to Luc's forceps, but difference is that it has no cutting edge and has simple joint instead of box joint in Luc's forceps.

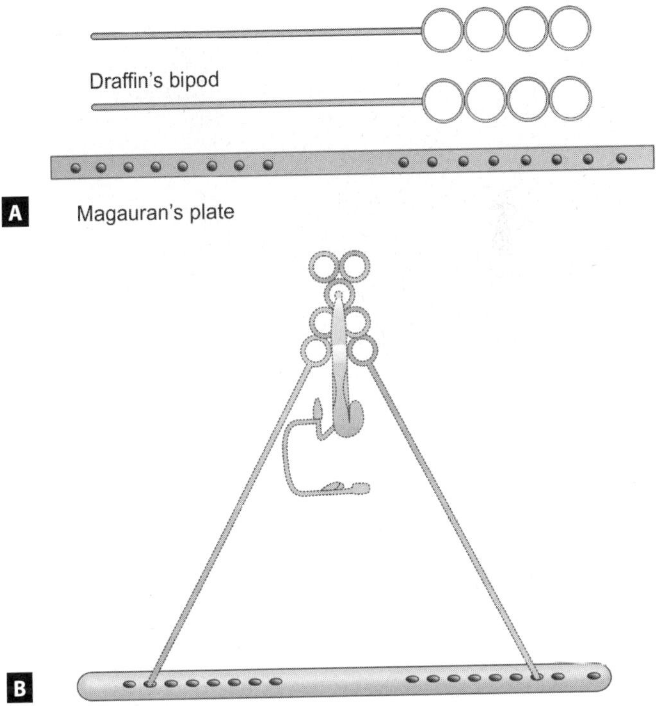

Figs 4.22A and B (A) Draffin's bipod and Magauran's plate; (B) Assembled mouth gag and tongue blade mounted on Magauran's plate

Waugh's Long Dissecting Forceps with Tooth (Fig. 4.25)

Used to put incision in tonsillectomy. Incision is put over the reflection of mucosa from tonsillar anterior pillar to tonsil, midway between upper pole and lower pole.

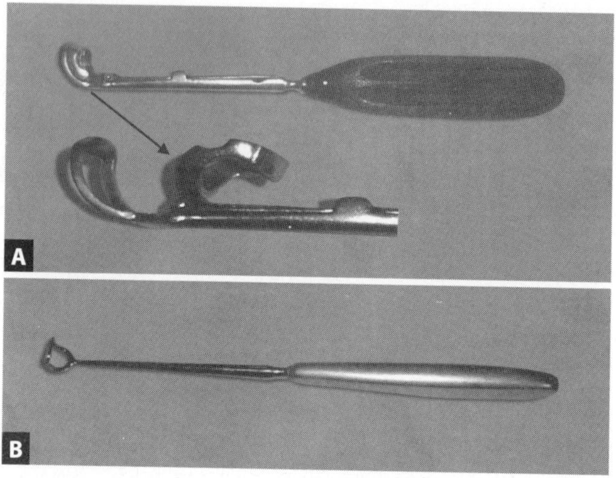

Figs 4.23A and B St Clair Thomson adenoid curette with (A) without guard (B)

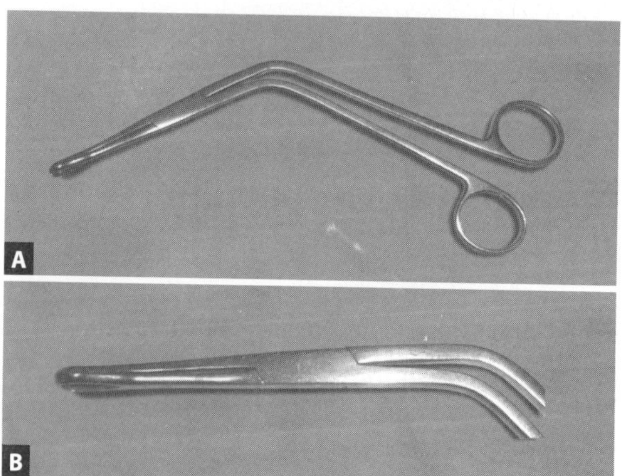

Figs 4.24A and B Denis Brown Tonsil holding forceps

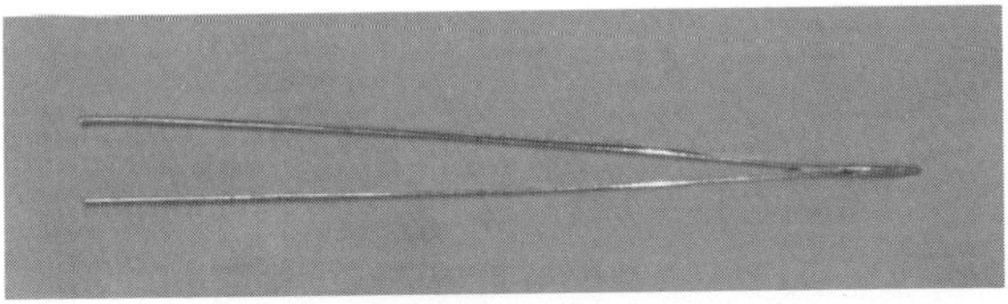

Fig. 4.25 Waugh's tenaculum forceps

Mollison's Tonsillar Dissector Cum Anterior Pillar Retractor (Fig. 4.26)

Uses:

- Dissecting end is used to divide the mucosa close to anterior pillar to expose the capsule and to dissect the tonsil from capsule down to the base of tonsil with minimal trauma
- Retracting end is used to retract the anterior pillar.

Yankauer's Pharyngeal Suction (Fig. 4.27)

Used to suck blood and secretions in tonsillectomy, adenoidectomy and all other oral and pharyngeal surgeries.

Eve's Tonsillar Snare (Fig. 4.28)

Used in tonsillectomy to snare the lower pole of tonsil. Advantage is that it crushes and then cut the tissue. On crushing, thromboplastin is released which is a vasoconstrictor. So bleeding is reduced.

Structures passing through lower pole of tonsil are:

- Triangular fold of tonsil
- Dorsal linguae vessel
- Lymphatics.

Negus Knot Pusher (Fig. 4.29)

Used to slip the ligature over tip of artery forceps in tonsillectomy (this should not be confused with Ballenger's swivel knife).

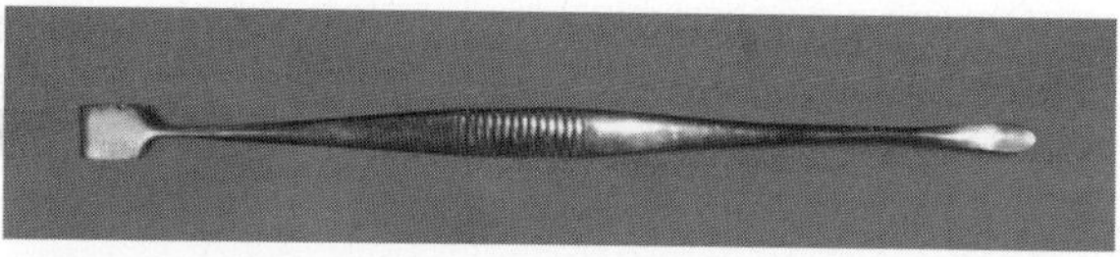

Fig. 4.26 Mollison's tonsillar dissector cum anterior pillar retractor

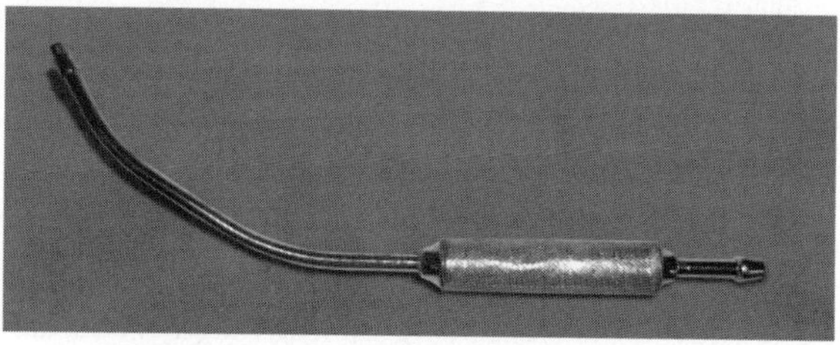

Fig. 4.27 Yankauer's pharyngeal suction

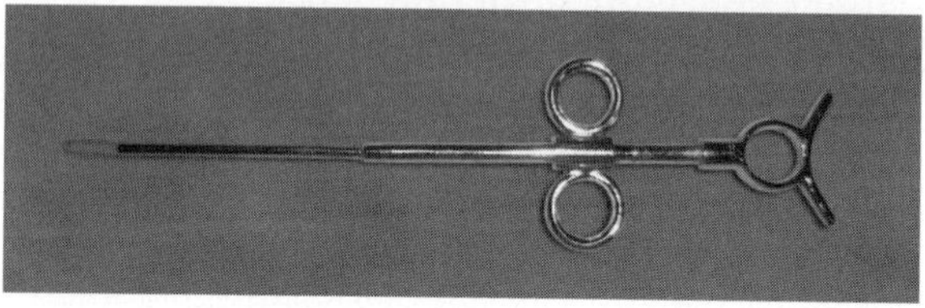

Fig. 4.28 Eve's tonsillar snare

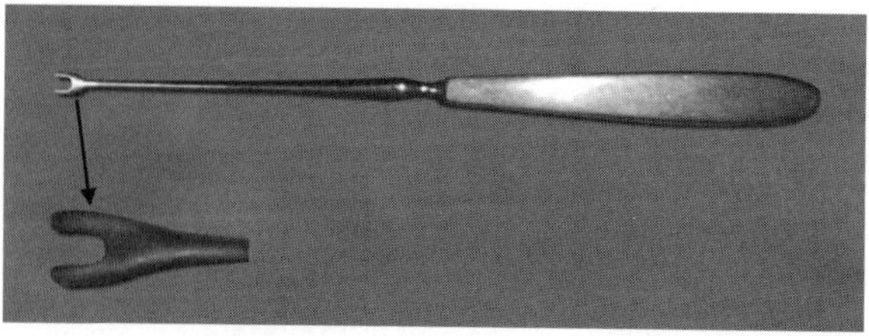

Fig. 4.29 Negus Knot pusher

Negus Tonsil Artery Forceps, Straight and Curved (Fig. 4.30)

To catch hold the bleeding vessel.

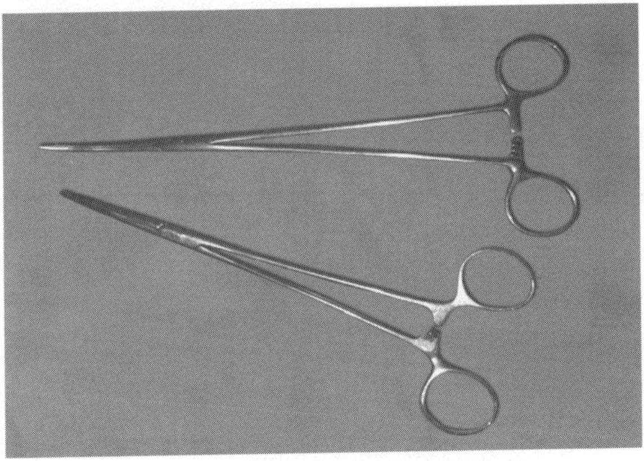

Fig. 4.30 Negus artery forceps

TRACHEOSTOMY TUBES

Various types are available.

- *Cuffed and uncuffed tubes:* Inflatable cuff prevents aspiration of blood and pharyngeal secretions. Prevent leakage of ventilating gases during anesthesia.
- Tubes made of silicon is preferred to German silver. Silicon causes less mucosal trauma and more flexibility than metal tubes.
- *Fenestrated tubes:* Fenestration allow air to pass through the tube and up through the larynx and this allows phonation. Tube of choice in children.

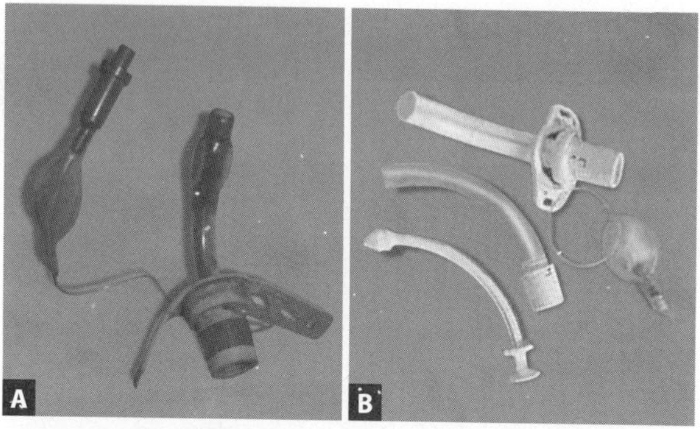

Figs 4.31A and B (A) Portex cuffed tube; (B) Shiley tube

- *Adjustable flang long tube:* Used to bypass a growth or stenosis of trachea.
  a. **Metallic tracheostomy tubes**
     - Jackson's tracheostomy tube
     - Fuller's tracheostomy tube.
  b. **Nonmetallic tracheostomy tubes**
     - Portex tracheostomy tube (Cuffed and uncuffed) **(Fig. 3.31A)**
     - Shiley tube **(Fig. 3.31B)**
  c. **Pediatric tracheostomy tubes**
     - Shiley tube
     - Alder Hey tube
     - Franklin tube of great ormond street.

Jackson's Metallic Tracheostomy Tube (Figs 4.32A and B)

Parts

Outer tube, inner tube, obturator.

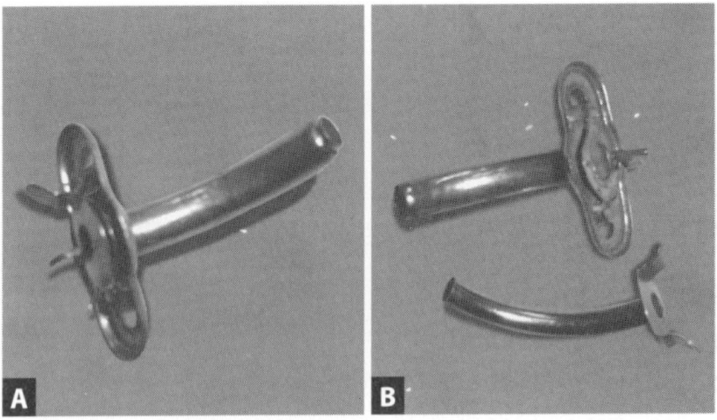

Figs 4.32A and B Jackson's metallic tracheostomy tube showing inner and outer tube

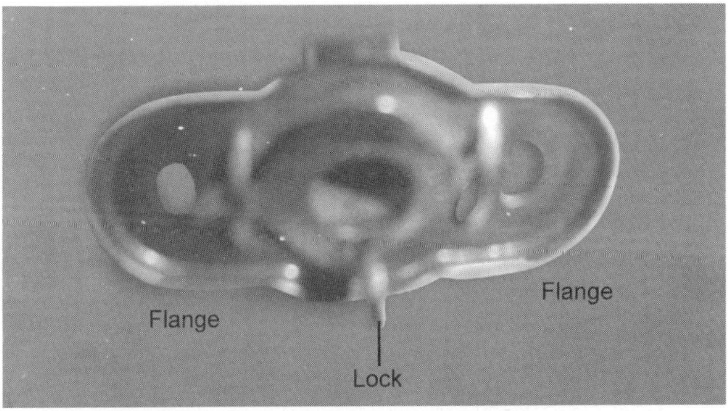

Fig. 4.33 Outer tube of Jackson's tracheostomy tube showing flanges and lock

Advantages

- Inner tube is longer than outer tube. This prevent obstruction of outer tube by secretion. Inner tube can be taken out and cleaned without disturbing the patency of main tracheostomy
- Outer tube has lock mechanism **(Fig. 4.33)**. This prevent the inner tube from falling out during cough.

- Obturator acts as pilot to dilate trachea while introducing tracheostomy tube
- Outer tube has flanges on both sides by which tube can be fixed to skin of neck.

Fuller's Tracheostomy Tube (Figs 4.34A and B)

Parts

Outer tube—biflanged tube
Inner tube—has an opening in the wall.

Advantages

- As outer tube is biflanged, size can be reduced by compressing the tube. This help in easy introduction
- Opening in the inner tube help in phonation (speech) during decannulation.

Disadvantages

- Tip of tube is sharp, so chance of being an irritant
- Flanges are weak, so chance of breaking is high
  This tube is used only at the time of decannulation.

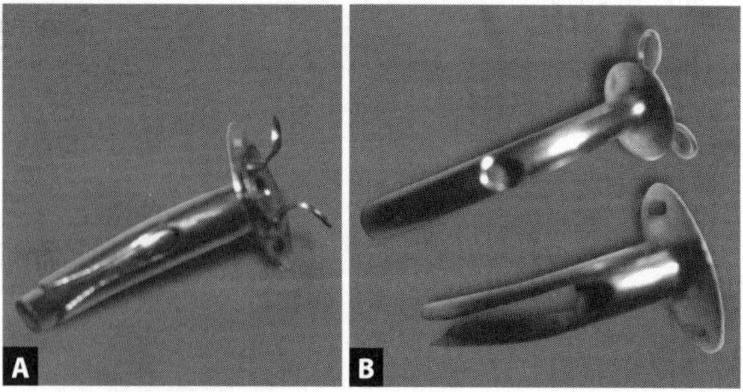

Figs 4.34A and B Fuller's tracheostomy tube

Nonmetallic Tracheostomy Tubes

- Used at the time of radiotherapy (Byproduct formed from the metal during radiation is toxic to lower respiratory tract. So, metallic tube is not used in RT).
- In permanent tracheostomy to prevent irritation, nonmetallic tube like Shiley tube is preferred
- Metallic tube are made of German silver. Nonmetallic are made of latex/polyvinyl chloride.

RIGID ENDOSCOPES

Jackson's Direct Laryngoscope (Fig. 4.35)

Use: For visualization of larynx and hypopharynx.

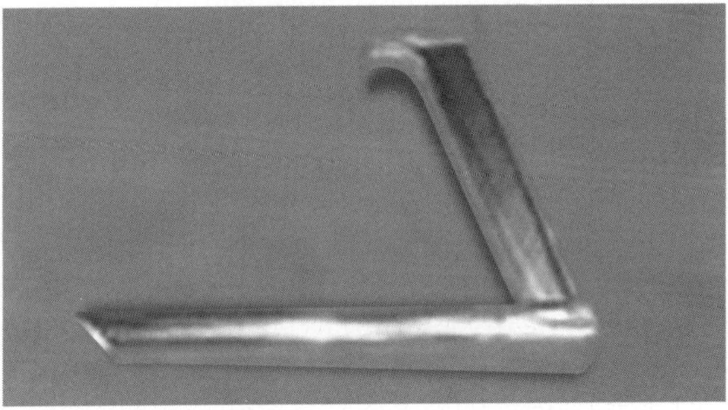

Fig. 4.35 Jackson's laryngoscope

Indications

- *Diagnostic:*
  - In situations where indirect laryngoscopy is difficult (excessive gag or overhanging epiglottis) or not possible

(infants and children). Nowadays, this indication is outdated because of availability of 70° scopes or flexible laryngoscope.
   - For taking biopsy from lesions larynx/hypopharynx
- *Therapeutic:*
   - Removal of benign lesions of larynx (papilloma, fibroma, etc.)
   - Removal of FB larynx and pharynx
   - Dilatation of laryngeal strictures.

Contraindications

- Diseases or injuries of cervical spine
- Recent coronary occlusion/cardiac decompensation
- Medical contraindications for surgery.

Q 1. How will you do direct laryngoscopy?

Ans: Can be done under LA/GA (GA is preferred). Position is Boyce position. Teeth protected with tooth guard. Laryngoscope lubricated with xylocaine gel held in left hand. Right hand is used to guide the laryngoscope and to hold suction and instruments. Laryngoscope introduced by one side of tongue. See the base of tongue and tip of epiglottis. Lift the epiglottis and advance laryngoscope. It gives good view of interior of larynx. If using anterior commissure laryngoscope its tip can be advanced further between the ventricular bands to examine the ventricle and anterior commissure.

Complications

- Injury to lips/tongue/teeth
- Bleeding
- Laryngeal edema/stridor.

Hypopharyngoscope (Fig. 4.36)

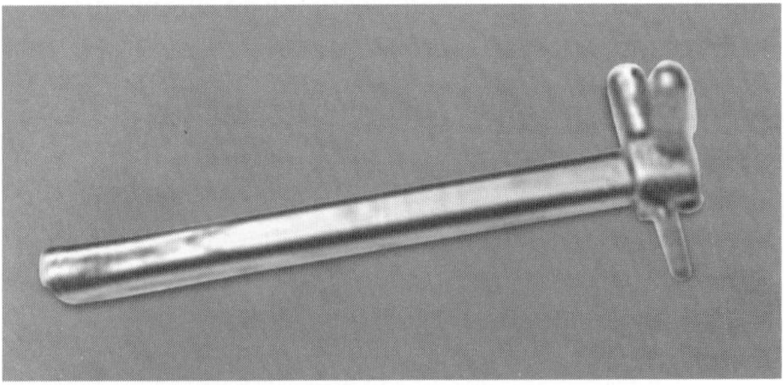

Fig. 4.36 Jackson's hypopharyngoscope

Length is 29 cm used to remove FB hypopharynx or to take biopsy in suspected malignancy.

Esophagoscope

Both rigid and fiberoptic scopes are available.

Jackson's Rigid Esophagoscope **(Fig. 4.37)**

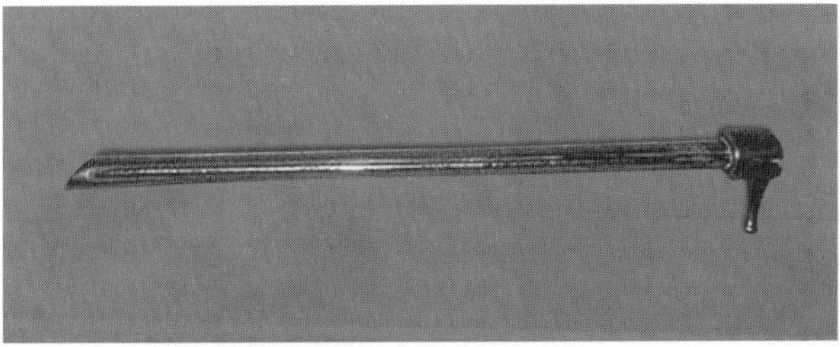

Fig. 4.37 Jackson's rigid esophagoscope

Q1. Name two rigid esophagoscopes.

Ans:

- Chevalier Jackson's esophagoscope (distal illumination)
- Fuller's esophagoscope (proximal illumination).

Q2. What are the indications of esophagoscopy?

Ans:

- *Diagnostic indications:*
  - As a part of investigation of dysphagia
  - To visualize any FB, stricture, growth esophagus
  - To take biopsy from esophageal lesion.
- *Therapeutic indications:*
  - Removal of FB esophagus
  - For dilatation of esophageal strictures, to pass Bougies
  - Sclerotherapy of esophageal varices.

Q3. What are the difference between Jackson and Negus esophagoscopes?

Ans: For Jackson esophagoscope, illumination is distal. So better clarity of field of vision. In Fuller's scope, it is proximal illumination [Chevalier Jackson—distal (remember as CD)].

Q4. How will you do esophagoscopy?

Ans:

Position: Boyce position (barking dog position/sniffing the morning air position), i.e. flexion of neck over chest and extension at atlantoaxial joint.

Technique: Tooth protected with tooth guard. Hold the esophagoscope vertically in right hand in pen holding fashion. Support the distal end (near mouth) with left hand. Advance esophagoscope through oral cavity on the right side of tongue, pharynx and right pyriform fossa till cricopharynx is visualized. Under general anesthesia, cricopharyngeal sphincter is relaxed and instrument is gently advanced. Introduce scope only after seeing the lumen. On reaching, midthorax tip of scope is advanced towards left anterior superior iliac spine.

Q5. What are the techniques to open the cricopharyngeal sphincter?

Ans:

- Apply persistent pressure with tip of scope to the crico-pharyngeal sphincter
- Apply 4% xylocaine to the sphincter and apply pressure
- Pass Ryle's tube first and then pass oscope.

Q6. What is the length of esophagus?

Ans: 25 cm.

Q7. How many constrictions? Name the site.

Ans: 4 constrictions.

- Cricopharynx—15 cm from upper lateral incisor
- Arch of aorta—25 cm from upper lateral incisor
- Left bronchus—28 cm from upper lateral incisor
- Diaphragm—40 cm from upper lateral incisor.

Q8. Curvatures of esophagus?

Ans: Two side-to-side curvatures both towards left. One at the root of neck and other at the lower end. Anteroposterior curvatures correspond to cervicothoracic spine.

Q9. What are the complications of rigid esophagoscopy?

Ans:

- Anesthesia complication
  - Aspiration
  - Arrhythmia
- Bleeding
- Cervical spine injury
- Pneumothorax
- Rupture of aortic aneurysm
- Esophageal perforation
- Trauma to lips and teeth.

The most common and most dreaded complication is perforation. Cervical esophagus at the level of cricopharynx is the most common site.

Q10. What are the clinical features of esophageal perforation?
Ans: Patient complaints severe pain interscapular area. On examination, there will be fall in blood pressure, tachycardia and emphysema at interscapular area.

Q11. What is the treatment of esophageal perforation?
Ans:

- Stop the procedure
- If esophagoscope in position, can introduce nasogastric tube. once withdrawn never put nasogastric (NG) tube blindly as there is chance of it going to peritoneal cavity
- Nil per oral and total parenteral nutrition
- High dose of broad-spectrum antibiotics
- High dose of parenteral steroids
- Correction of fluid and electrolyte imbalance
- If patient not improving with conservative treatment or if large perforation, surgical repair of perforation is needed. Do left lateral pharyngotomy for cervical esophageal perforation repair. *Best time for repair is within 6 hours of perforation.*

Q12. What are the contraindications of this scopy?
Ans:

- Trismus
- Diseases of cervical spine (Cervical trauma, spondylosis, kyphosis)
- Aneurysm of aorta for fear of rupture and fatal hemorrage.

Bronchoscope

Both rigid and fiberoptic scopes are available.

Rigid Bronchoscope (*Fig. 4.38*)

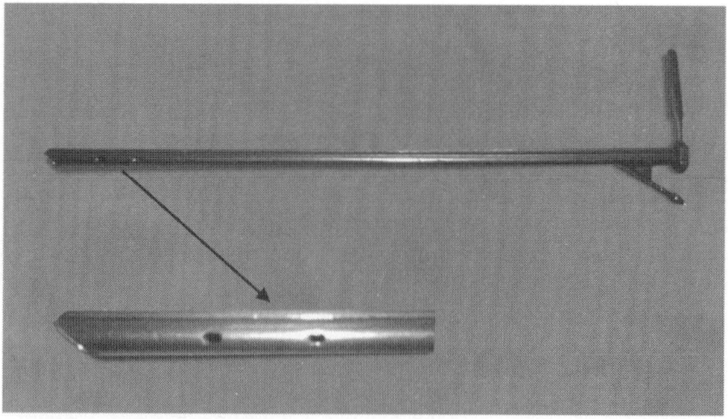

Fig. 4.38 Jackson's rigid bronchoscopes showing ventilation holes

Q. What are the indications?

Ans:

- *Diagnostic:*
  - To take biopsy from suspected lesions
  - As part of panendoscopy
  - To find out cause for wheezing, hemoptysis or unexplained cough persisting for more than 4 weeks.
- *Theraputic:*
  - For removal of FB bronchus
  - For bronchial aspiration in case of lung abscess and aspiration pneumonia.

Procedure done preferably under general anesthesia (Apneic technique/Jet ventilation).

Difference between right esophagoscope and bronchoscope is given in **Table 4.1**.

Endotracheal Tubes (Fig. 4.39)

- Made of latex/PVC/rubber/silicone
- Radius of curvature from 12–16 cm
- Tube internal and external diameters should be circular

Table 4.1 Difference between rigid esophagoscope and bronchoscope

Esophagoscope	*Bronchoscope*
• Longer with wider lumen • Has markings on the scope • Tip is smooth and blunt • No ventilation holes on side	• Shorter with narrow lumen • No markings • Tip is sharp • Ventilation holes on side

Markings on esophagoscope are to locate the tip of scope
Side ventilation holes in bronchoscope are to ventilate the opposite bronchus
Carina is the first endobronchial landmark during bronchoscopy

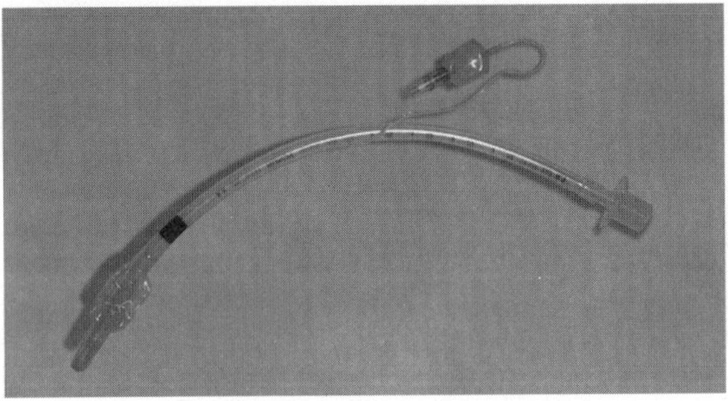

Fig. 4.39 Cuffed endotracheal tubes

- Murphy eye is the hole through the tube opposite to the bevel. Purpose of the eye is to provide an alternate pathway for the gas flow, if the bevel is blocked.
- Blue line is the radiopaque marker placed along the whole length of the tube for determination of position of tube radiologically after intubation.
- Cuffed and uncuffed tubes are available.

Q: What are the advantages of cuffed tubes?

Ans:

- Improved monitoring
- Absence of leak during ventillation

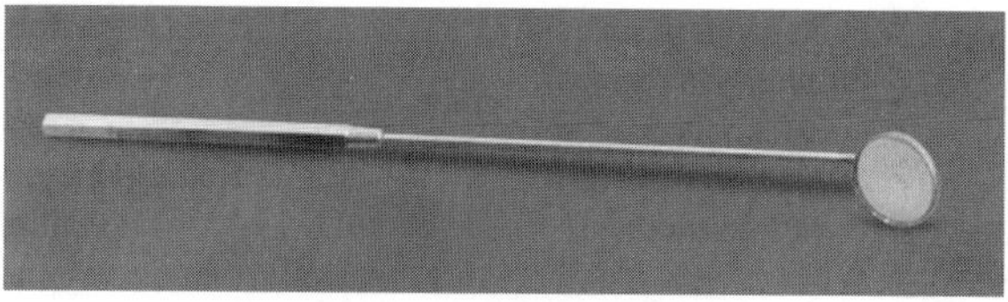

Fig. 4.40 Laryngeal mirror

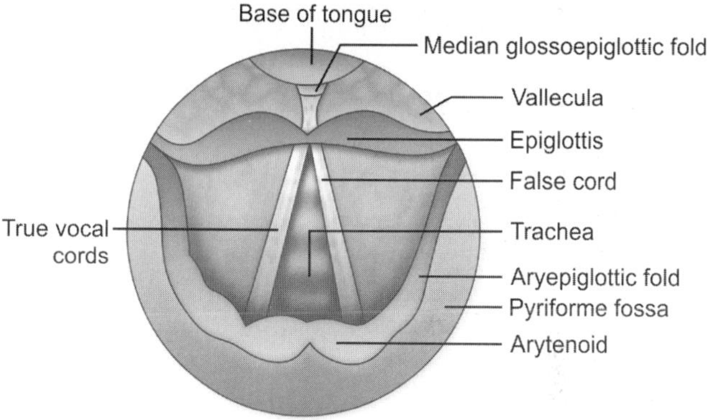

Fig. 4.41 Indirect laryngoscopy

Table 4.2 Difference between direct and indirect laryngoscopy

Indirect laryngoscopy	*Direct laryngoscopy*
• Operative procedure, less morbidity	• Operative procedure
• Done using laryngeal mirror	• Done using direct laryngoscope
• Image seen is virtual	• Real image
• Foreshortening of AP diameter of image	• Actual length of vocal cords seen
• Blind areas difficult to see	• Whole area exposed
• Diagnostic procedure	• Both diagnostic and therapeutic

- Ability to use positive end expiratory pressure (PEEP)
  - Narrowest part of adult airway is *glottis*
  - Narrowest part of child's airway is *subglottis*.

Laryngeal Mirror (Fig. 4.40)

Used to do indirect laryngoscopic examination **(Fig. 4.41 and Table 4.2)**.

Q. What are the blind areas on indirect laryngoscopy?

Ans:

- Laryngeal surface of epiglottis
- Ventricle
- Anterior commissure
- Subglottis
- Postcricoid area
- Apex of pyriform fossa.

CHAPTER 5

Operative Surgery in ENT

EAR

Myringotomy

Making an opening in tympanic membrane (TM) (myringus=tympanic membrane).

Q1. Write five indications of myringotomy.

Ans:

1. Acute suppurative otitis media-buldging TM with impending rupture, severe ear pain or with suspected complications despite adequate antibiotic treatment.
2. Secretory otitis media (SOM).
3. Aero-otitis media.
4. Atelectasis ear.
5. Meniere's disease.

Q2. What are the types of incisions for myringotomy?

Ans: **Figure 5.1**.

A. Radial incision in anteroinferior quadrant in serous otitis media for ventilating middle ear.
B. J-shaped circumferential incision in posteroinferior quadrant in acute suppurative otitis media.

Q3. Why radial incision in SOM?

Ans: In radial incision, edges get better approximation and will hold the ventilation tube in place. In circular incision, blood supply from annulus is cut off, not in radial incision.

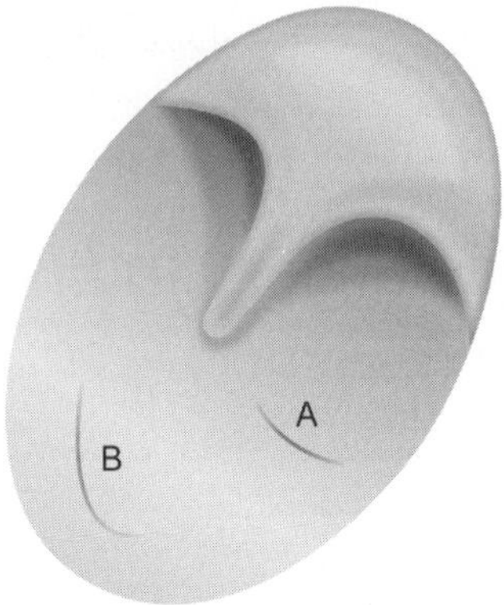

Fig. 5.1 Myringotomy incisions

Q4. What is the purpose of putting ventilation tubes in SOM?
Ans: Ventilation tubes establish adequate aeration of middle ear cleft, with consequent reversion of pathological changes of middle ear mucosa.

Q5. What are the complications of myringotomy?
Ans:
- Injury to incudostapedial joint
- Injury to chorda tympani nerve
- Middle ear infection
- Injury to jugular bulb, if high jugular bulb or floor of middle ear is dehiscent
- Permanent perforation of TM and tympanosclerosis is a late complication.

Surgeries on Mastoid

It includes:
- *Myringoplasty:* Surgical procedure involving simple repair of tympanic membrane perforation in which no ossicular reconstruction is involved.

- *Tympanoplasty:* Surgical procedure which includes, *eradication* of disease from tympanic cavity, *reconstruction* of hearing apparatus, *with/without* tympanic membrane grafting and *without* mastoid exploration.
- *Mastoid exploration:* Includes *canal wall up* procedures and *canal wall down* procedures.

  Canal wall up procedures:
  1. Cortical mastoidectomy
  2. Combined approach tympanoplasty (CAT).

  Canal wall down procedures:
  1. Radical mastoidectomy
  2. Modified radical mastoidectomy (MRM)
  3. Atticotomy (epitympanotomy)
  4. Attico antrostomy (epitympanomastoidectomy/Bondy's mastoidectomy).
- Mastoid obliteration.

Approaches to Mastoid

Postaural Incision of William Wilde ***(Fig. 5.2)***

Starts from highest attachment of pinna up to tip of mastoid 0.5–1 cm behind postaural groove. *In infants and children up to 2 years of age, mastoid process is not developed and facial nerve lies exposed near exit from stylomastoid foramen. So, incision is more horizontal.*

Advantages

- Excellent, wide exposure of mastoid aircells and epitympanum and allows access to posterior fossa
- Cosmetically appealing
- Easy to perform.

Endaural Incision by Lempert ***(Fig. 5.3)***

It consist of two parts:

1. *Lempert-I:* Semicircular incision made from 12 o'clock to 6 o'clock position in the posterior meatal wall at bony cartilaginous junction

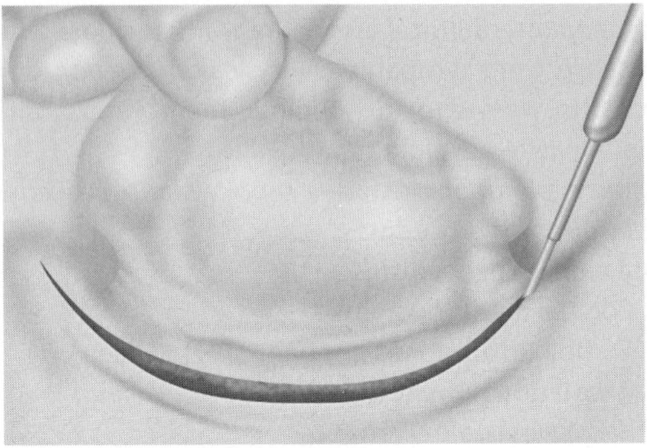

Fig. 5.2 William Wilde postaural incision

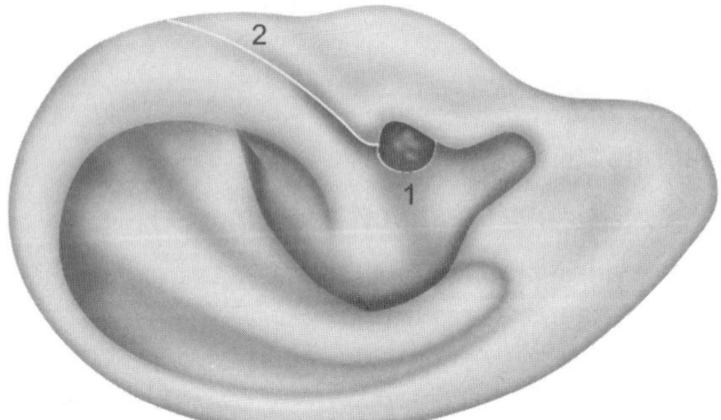

Fig. 5.3 Endaural incision

2. *Lempert-II:* Starts from 1st incision at 12 o'clock and then passes upwards in a curvilinear fashion through incisura terminalis (between tragus and crus of helix).

Advantages

- Provides direct head on access to the mesotympanum, epitympanum, aditus and antrum and external osseous meatus

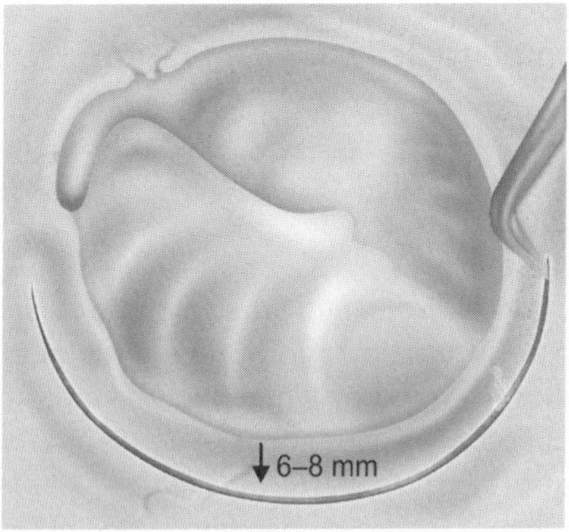

Fig. 5.4 Transcanal incision

- Incision is made in the cartilage-free gap. So, chance of perichondritis is minimal
- Both mastoid and external canal surgery can be done by this incision.

Disadvantages

- Tendency for stenosis formation at the bony cartilaginous junction of external auditory canal
- Difficulty in gaining access to mastoid tip cells.

Endomeatal/Transcanal Incision by Rosen ***(Fig. 5.4)***

The best approach for exploration of middle ear cleft. It is a bucket handle type of incision made in the posterior canal skin, extending from the 12 o'clock position superiorly to the 6 o'clock position inferiorly, and curving outward to the level of isthmus at its midpoint. This incision *should not* be attempted in the presence of either diffuse or localized external otitis.

- Position for all ear surgeries is supine with operated ear up (head turned to operated side)
- Anesthesia can be GA/LA.

Cortical Mastoidectomy (Simple/Complete/Schwartz Operation)

Indications

- CSOM TTD ACTIVE not responding to adequate course of appropriate antibiotic
- Masked mastoiditis
- *Acute coalescent mastoiditis:* When symptoms and signs have not been controlled by appropriate antibiotic/or presence of complications/and or when acute symptoms and signs subside but otorrhea continues 3–4 weeks after onset.
- As an approach *to perform cochlear implant surgery,* endolymphatic sac surgery, decompression of facial nerve.

Steps

- Incision described above. Incision deepened. Periosteum cut and elevated identify MacEwen's triangle
  - Boundaries of MacEwen's triangle are superior temporal line superiorly, posterior bony canal wall anteriorly and a tangent drawn to canal wall posteriorly. It is the surgical land mark for mastoid antrum which usually lies 2–2.5 cm deep to it.
- *Removal of mastoid cortex and exposure of antrum:* Drill cortical bone with mastoid drill and largest size cutting burr.
  - Commonly in use is a micromotor drill. Other types of drills are hanging and table top type.
  - *Korners septum:* Persistent petrosquamous lamina which can be misdiagnosed as mastoid antrum.
  - Mastoid antrum is identified by seeing the aditus in its anterior wall and lateral semicircular canal in its medial wall.
- Removal of all accessible air cells.

- Widening of aditus ad antrum (connection between middle ear and mastoid, lies at superomedial wall of mastoid antrum) and establishing adequate drainage.
- Closure of wound in layers and mastoid dressings applied.

Postoperative Care

- Soon after recovery from anesthesia, facial movements are examined to exclude damage to facial nerve
- Antibiotic therapy for one week
- Stitch removed after 5–6 days.

Complications

- Persistent deafness
- Injury to facial nerve
- Injury to horizontal semicircular canal
- Dislocation of incus
- Injury to sigmoid sinus/dura
- Postoperative wound infection and wound break down
  - In a completed complete mastoidectomy, cavity having bevelled edges with bony plate of tegmen tympani above, sinus plate behind, inferiorly mastoid tip and anteriorly to the limit of pneumatization in posterior root of zygoma
  - Persistent discharge after surgery is due to
    1. Operation performed too early, before localization of infection
    2. Incomplete removal of mastoid air cells
    3. Presence of petrositis
    4. Erroneously performed for allergic otitis media or for cholesteatoma.

Radical Mastoidectomy

Indications

- Unresectable cholesteatoma extending down the Eustachian tube or into petrous apex
- Promontory cochlear fistula caused by cholesteatoma
- Chronic perilabrynthine cholestatoma/ostitis that cannot be removed
- Resection of temporal bone neoplasm with periodic monitoring.

Steps

- Incision
- Exposure of macEwen's triangle
- Exposure of mastoid antrum and exenteration of all accessible air cells
- Removal of bridge (bridge is part of posterior canal wall which overlies aditus)
- Lowering of ridge (part of posterior bony canal wall which overlies vertical part of facial nerve
- *Toilet of middle ear:* Remnants of tympanic membrane with its annulus and sulcus tympanicus is removed. Malleus, incus and middle ear mucoperiosteum removed. Stapes left intact. Eustachian tube opening is permanently closed. Also removal of cholesteatoma/granulation tissue
- Meatoplasty
- Closure of wound
- Structures removed in radical mastoidectomy (RM)
  - Malleus
  - Incus
  - Middle ear mucosa
  - Remnants of TM.

Postoperative Care

Dressings, antibiotics, cavity care.

Complications

- Facial paralysis
- Injury to dura/sigmoid sinus
- Perichondritis pinna
- Cavity problems - 4D - Deafness
Discharge
Dizziness
Dependence
- Mucous cyst.

Modified Radical Mastoidectomy

Indication

CSOM-AAD cholesteatoma/granulation tissue middle ear/mastoid.

Differences between Radical and Modified Radical Mastoidectomy

- Here we remove only diseased tissue (cholesteatoma/ granulation tissue/unhealthy mucosa are removed)
- Healthy ossicles and tympanic membrane remnants are preserved
- Hearing mechanism is reconstructed in modified radical mastoidectomy (MRM).

Myringoplasty

Prerequisites

- Dry ear for atleast 3–6 weeks
- Eustachian tube should be functioning normally

- Ossicular chain should be intact
- All predisposing factors treated adequately/no focus of infection in nose, PNS and nasopharynx
- Adequate cochlear reserve (no sensorineural hearing loss)
- Perforation should be central without presence of cholesteatoma.

Indications

- *Auditory:* Closure of perforation for improving hearing and decreasing tinnitus
- *Protection:* Protects middle ear from recurrent infection
- To enable proper fitting hearing aid
- To enable recruitment in certain professions.

Contraindications

- Presence of cholesteatoma in ear
- Perforation in only hearing ear
- Medical contraindication for surgery.

Techniques

Two grafting techniques:

- *Overlay:* Graft placed lateral to tympanic membrane
- *Underlay:* Graft placed medial to tympanic membrane.

Complications

Overlay technique

- Anterior angle blunting (anterior blunting)
- Epithelial pearls
- Graft lateralization
- Prolonged healing.

Underlay technique

- Narrowing of middle ear
- Graft may get adhered to promontory
- Anterior perforation.

Results are better with underlay technique as compared with overlay.

Other procedures for closure of tympanic membrane perforation:

- Cauterization—50% trichloracetic acid, phenol
- Splinting of traumatic perforations
- Closure by prosthesis like paper disk moistened with 1% phenol in glycerine.

Materials used for grafting in myringoplasty

- Temporalis fascia, the most common graft material because
  - Ease of harvest from same incision as the operation
  - Availability of large amount of graft
  - Very high take rate without subsequent problems
- Tragal perichondrium
- Fascia lata
- Porcine dura and calf jugular vein (xenograft)
- Cadaveric dura (not preferred as possibility of transmission of prion vector disease such as Creutzfeldt-Jakob encephalopathy.

Tympanoplasty

Definition given above.

Types of tympanoplasty (by Wolfstein):

- Myringoplasty with restoration of normal middle ear
- Ossiculoplasty
- Myringostapediopexy
- Round window baffling (RW protection)
- Fenestration of horizontal semicircular canal.

Contraindications

- Malignant neoplasms of outer/middle ear
- Invasive, life-threatening *Pseudomonas* infection of ear
- Intracranial complications of ear diseases
- Medical contraindications for surgery
- Only hearing ear.

Prosthesis in use for Ossiculoplasty

- *TORP:* Total ossicular replacement prosthesis
- *PORP:* Partial ossicular replacement prosthesis
- Plastipore
- Proplast
- Teflon.

Stapedectomy

Treatment of choice for otosclerosis (other treatment option is hearing aid fitting):

- Usually done under local anesthesia. Can be done under general anesthesia (GA)
- Permeatal/transcanal incision
- Elevate tympanomeatal flap
- Preserve/cut chorda tympani nerve
- Bony overhang of posterior canal wall removed
- Ossicles are palpated with a probe and stapedial fixation confirmed
- Stapedius tendon cut, incudostapedial joint disarticulated
- Removal of stapes suprastructure
- Creation of fenestra in footplate
- *Piston placement:* Piston hooked around long process of incus and fitted in the hole made in footplate
- Replace tympanomeatal flap. External auditory cana (EAC) packed with gelfoam.

Complications

- Injury to chora tympani/facial nerve
- Hemotympanum
- Tear of TM
- Perilymph fistula
- Labrynthitis
- Sensorinural hearing loss
- Acute otitis media
- Necrosis of long process of incus and slipping of prosthesis
- Postoperative granuloma.

Contraindications

- Only hearing ear
- Young children, professional athlets, divers, etc.
- Otitis externa, TM perforation and exostosis are relative contraindications.

NOSE

Position: Reverse Trendelenberg with 15° neck flexion. Advantage is that better visualization of nasal cavity and less venous congestion, so that chance of bleeding is less.

Caldwell-Luc Operation (Radical Sublabial Antrostomy)

It is a surgical procedure containing three main steps:

1. *Sublabial incision*: Starting from canine ridge to 1st molar tooth
2. *Anterior maxillotomy*: Opening of the anterior wall and intra-antral inspection and manipulation
3. *Inferior meatal antrostomy*: Maxillary antrum connected to nose through nasoantral window made in inferior meatus.

Q1. What are the indications?

Ans: **COFFEE BOARD**

C **C**hronic sinusitis
O **O**roantral fistula
F **F**ungal sinusitis
F **F**oreign body maxilla [common foreign body (FB) are dental amalgam and bullet]
E **E**thmoidectomy (Transantral ethmoidectomy-Jansen Horgan procedure)
E **E**levation of orbital floor fracture (here Caldwel approach is used)
B ***B**iopsy:* Excision biopsy of benign lesions of maxilla. For malignancy biopsy by this approach is not preferred as it leads to spread of neoplasm to cheek
O **T**o make opening on posterior wall of maxilla (as in maxillary artery ligation, vidian neurectomy)
A **A**ntrochoanal polyp
R **R**eduction fracture maxilla
D **D**entigerous cyst.

Q2. What are the contraindications?

Ans:

1. Hypoplasia maxilla
2. Bleeding disorders
3. Children as chance of damage to secondary dentition.

Q3. What are the complications?

Ans:

1. Anesthesia cheek due to stretching of infraorbital nerve
2. Anesthesia teeth
3. Injury to nasolacrimal duct
4. Oroantral fistula
5. Osteomyelitis of maxilla
6. Hemorrhage from branches of sphenopalatine artery.

Q4. Name a condition which is an indication and complication of Caldwell-Luc?

Ans: Oroantral fistula.

Q5. Postoperative care.

Ans:

1. Keep ice pack over cheek for 4–6 hours to prevent edema.
2. Avoid blowing of nose for 2 weeks.

Septoplasty

Repair of nasal septum. Classical approach is *Cottle's maxilla premaxila approach of septoplasty.*

Indications

1. Deviated nasal septum causing symptoms like nasal block, recurrent sinusitis, epistaxis and headache.
2. As part of septorrhinoplasty for cosmetic purpose.
3. *Nonseptal indications:* As approach to pituitary, prior to tympanoplasty, harvesting cartilage graft, etc.

Done in

- Anterior deviations; deviations anterior to *Cottle's line* (imaginary line drawn from nasal process of frontal bone to nasal spine of maxilla)
- In children under 18 years septoplasty is preferred to submucous resection (SMR).

Contraindications

- Acute infection of nose or sinus
- Medical contraindication for surgery
- Bleeding disorders.

Table 5.1 Differences between septoplasty and submucous resection (SMR)

Septoplasty	*SMR*
• *Incision:* Freer's incision • Elevation of mucoperichondrial flap on one side	• Killian incision (posterior incision) • Flap elevated on both sides
• Only deviated part of cartilage removed	• Entire cartilage, except a caudal and dorsal strut, removed
• Chance of complications minimal	• Complications more

Position: Described above.

Anesthesia: Local/general.

Infiltrate 2% xylocaine with 1: 1 lakh adrenaline into both side of nasal septum (adrenaline being a vasoconstrictor reduces bleeding, increases duration of action of xylocaine and reduces toxicity of xylocaine).

Incision: Freer's incision (curvilinear incision at caudal end of septal cartilage).

Elevate mucoperichondrial flap on one side. Separate septal cartilage from vomer and perpendicular plate of ethmoid and raise mucoperiosteal flap on both sides. Correct bony septum by removing deformed parts. Remove deviated part of septal cartilage. Remove maxillary crest to realign the septal cartilage. Put trans-septal sutures to coapt mucoperichondrial flaps and also suturing of incision. Nasal packing done.

See **Table 5.1** for differences between septoplasty and SMR.

Complications

Immediate

- Bleeding
- Damage to surrounding structures—injury to septal flap, turbinate
- Anesthesia complications.

Late

- Synachiae
- Septal hematoma
- Septal abscess
- Septal perforation
- Flapping of septum
- External deformities are more common with SMR
- Toxic shock syndrome—rare after septal surgery
  - External deformities seen after SMR
    - i. Saddle nose deformity
    - ii. Supratip deformity (Polly beak deformity)
    - iii. Retraction of columella.

Endoscopic Sinus Surgery

Indications

- Chronic bacterial sinusitis unresponsive to adequate dose of appropriate antibiotics. This is the absolute indication for functional endoscopic sinus surgery
- Fungal sinusitis with fungal ball
- Antrochoanal polyp
- Mucocele of any of the sinuses
- Control of epistaxis by endoscopic cauterization and artery ligation
- Repair of choanal atresia
- Removal of benign tumors like inverted papilloma/ angiofibroma
- Orbital conditions like dacryocystorhinostomy for chronic decryocystitis, optic nerve decompression
- Repair of CSF rhinorrhea and trans-sphenoidal hypophysectomy.

Contraindications/Limitations

- Diseases inaccessible by endoscopic surgery (lateral wall and floor of maxillary sinus, lateral recesses of frontal sinus, etc.)
- Threatened intracranial/intraorbital complications
- Inexperience and lack of proper instrumentation.

Anesthesia: LA/GA (hypotensive anesthesia is preferred).

Basic Steps

- Uncinectomy/infundibulotomy
- Middle meatal antrostomy
- Anterior ethmoidectomy/posterior ethmoidectomy/ sphenoidotomy/frontal recess clearance, as depending on involvement of sinus
- Clearance of disease.

Complications

- *Orbital:* Periorbital ecchymosis, emphysema, orbital hematoma, optic nerve injury, blindness (chance is more in posterior ethmoid and sphenoid sinus surgeries)
- *Intracranial:* Meningitis, CSF leak, direct injury to brain, Tension pneumocephalus, carotid artey injury
- Hemorrhage from sphenopalatine and ethmoid arteries
- Injury to nasolacrimal duct
- Anosmia
- Synechiae.

Tracheostomy

Indications

- To relieve respiratory obstruction which may be due to
  - *Trauma:* Laryngeal injury (due to acute trauma, inhalation of fumes, swallowing of corrosives) facial bone fractures, hematoma base of tongue

  - *Tumor:* Tumors of larynx and laryngopharynx/base of tongue both benign and malignant
  - Infection and inflammations due to diseases of respiratory tract like laryngeal diphtheria, acute laryngotracheal bronchitis, acute epiglottitis
  - Bilateral abductor paralysis of vocal cords
  - Impacted FB in larynx and trachea
  - *Congenital:* Laryngomalacia, subglottic stenosis, laryngeal web, etc.
- Retained secretions. As tracheal toilet—for taking out retained secretions from lower respiratory tract
  - Inability to cough-coma of any cause, paralysis of respiratory muscles, spasm of respiratory muscles as in tetanus
  - Painful cough-chest injuries
  - Aspiration of bronchial secretions as in bulbar polio
- Respiratory insufficiency
  - Chronic lung conditions—emphysema, chronic bronchitis.

Types of Tracheostomy

1. a. Elective
   b. Emergency
2. a. *High tracheostomy:* At the level of thyroid isthmus. Damages 1st tracheal ring. Only indication is carcinoma larynx, for which later planning for total laryngectomy. This can lead to subglottic stenosis.
   b. *Mid tracheostomy:* Preferred one. Done at the level of 2nd and 3rd tracheal ring.
   c. *Low tracheostomy:* Chance of damage to great vessels of neck and apical pleura especially in children. Elective low tracheostomy is done in stridor due to laryngeal trauma.

3. a. Temporary
   b. *Permanent:* Needed in bilateral abductor paralysis, laryngeal stenosis or in laryngectomy patients.

What are the advantages of tracheostomy over intubation?

1. Tracheostomy can be kept for longer period of time and easy to maintain
2. It decreases dead space by 80 mL
3. Tracheal toilet is easy
4. Greater comfort to the patient than intubation.

What are the functions of tracheostomy?

1. Act as alternate pathway for breathing
2. Improves alveolar ventilation by decreasing dead space by 30–40% and by reducing the resistance to airflow
3. Protects lower airways from aspiration of blood or pharyngeal secretions
4. Permits removal of tracheobronchial secretions
5. For giving IPPR (intermittent positive pressure ventilation)
6. To administer anesthesia in case of difficult intubation as in patients with trismus.

Position: Supine with extension of neck, so as to keep trachea anteriorly. Pillow kept under the shoulder and a head ring.

Anesthesia

- Local
- General
- Local after intubation (this is the safest one because intubation decreases intrathoracic pressure, so bleeding is reduced. It also decreases the chance of injury to neighboring structures like cervical pleura.

Incision

- Vertical
- Horizontal

Vertical incision: From lower border of cricoid cartilage to sternal notch in the midline of neck. It is easier, faster with less bleeding. This is ideal for emergency tracheostomy. Disadvantage is that it causes bad scar.

Horizontal incision: Between anterior border of two sternocledomastoid muscle, midway between cricoid cartilage and sternal notch. Scar is less with this but chance of bleeding is more.

Procedure

After incision tissues are dissected in the midline. Strap muscles separated in the midline and dissected laterally. Thyroid isthmus retracted upwards or ligated and cut. 4% xylocaine injected into tracheal lumen before putting tracheal incision. Before spraying withdraw needle to see air bubbles to confirm that needle is in the lumen. Make opening (vertical incision) in anterior wall of trachea in the region of 2nd and 3rd/3rd and 4th tracheal rings. Opening should be of optimum size. Tracheostomy tube of appropriate size is inserted and retained by tapes passed around neck.

There is chance of post-tracheostomy apnea due to wash out of CO_2 with rapid improvement of oxygenation after tracheostomy. Treatment is carbogen inhalation (carbogen is a mixture of 95% oxygen and 5% carbon dioxide). Rebreathing into polythene bag tied to tracheostomy opening is a practical solution.

Postoperative care of tracheostomy

- *Positioning of tube:* Proper attention for correct positioning of the tube by selecting proper size and securing it to neck.
- Tracheostomized patient cannot shout or call for help. So, a bell/nurse/paper and pen should be available to patient round the clock.
- *Suctioning of tracheostomy tube:* Inner tube should be cleaned and replaced every 2 hourly. Give frequent suction depending on amount of secretions. Outer tube should not be removed

for minimum 10 days. If using cuffed tube, cuff should be deflated for a period of 5 minutes in every one hour.

- *Humidification and prevention of crusting:* Dry air encourages crust formation and decreases ciliary action. Constant temperature of 70°F maintained with proper humidification. A boiling water kettle in the room provides humidifier air if no facilities for condenser humidifier or ultrasonic humidifier. If there is crusting, few drops of hypotonic saline/ringer lactate/5% sodium bicarbonate instilled into trachea to loosen crusts. Secretions removed from trachea and bronchi with soft sterile catheter.
- Antibiotics and supportive as needed.

Complications

Immediate

A. Apnea due to sudden decrease in CO_2
B. *Bleeding:* Anterior jugular vein and inferior thyroid veins are the common sites of bleeding also isthmus of thyroid gland
C. Cardiac failure
D. Damage of surrounding structures (recurrent laryngeal nerve, esophagus)
E. Emphysema (surgical emphysema).

Intermediate

Dislodgement of tube, blocked tube, tracheitis, subcutaneous emphysema, bleeding, tracheovenous fistula, pneumothorax.

Late

Tracheocutaneous fistula, tracheal stenosis, laryngeal stenosis, difficult decannulation (the most common long-term complication in children).

Causes of Difficult Decannulation

- Persistence of condition for which tracheostomy was done

- Granulation tissue around stoma (peristomal and suprastomal granulations)
- Edema tracheal mucosa
- Psychological dependence
- Tracheomalacia
- Subglottic stenosis.

Differences between Adult and Infant Tracheostomy

- Trachea in infants and children is soft and compressible than adult. So, identification is difficult
- Trachea is simply incised without removing piece of tracheal wall in children
- Tracheal lumen is small in children, so chance of injury to posterior tracheal wall or esophagus is more in children than in adult.

Adenoidectomy

What are the methods of adenoidectomy?

Ans:

- Transoral curettage (Traditional method)
- Endoscopic adenoidectomy with forceps, suction diathermy and microdebrider.

Indication

Adenoid hypertrophy causing bilateral nasal block with rhinolalia clausa (hyponasality), obstructive sleep apnea syndrome, recurrent rhinosinusitis, secretory otitis media and failure to thrive.

Contraindications

- Cleft palate/submucous cleft palate (removal of adenoid will cause velopharyngeal insufficiency in these)
- Acute respiratory infection
- Bleeding disorders.

Anesthesia: GA-orotracheal intubation.

Position: Rose's position (supine with extension of neck over chest by placing a sand bag under shoulder, a head ring to stabilize the head).

Steps

- Open mouth using Boyle-Davis mouth gag and Daughty's tongue blade.
- Palpate nasopharynx digitally to confirm size of adenoid and also to medialize lateral adenoid tissue. Curetting the lateral adenoid tissue over Eustachian cushion area can cause scarring and permanent middle ear problems.
- Proper size St Clair Thompson adenoid curette with guard is introduced into nasopharynx. Introduce till it touches posterior end of nasal septum and engage in adenoid tissue. With sweeping movement of wrist joint of right hand curette out the adenoid mass. *While curetting use left hand to flex the neck of patient.* This is to avoid injury to anterior spinal ligament and odontoid process.
- Keep a gauze pack in nasopharynx to get hemostasis. Usually pack is kept for just more than the clotting time of patient.

Complications

- *Bleeding:* The most common cause is adenoid remnant. Removal of remnant usally controls bleeding. If not stopped keep postnasal pack for 24–48 hours
- Injury to Eustachian tube opening
- Velopharyngeal insufficiency
- Recurrence
- *Grisel's syndrome:* While curetting adenoids, due to inadvertent exposure of anterior spinal ligament there is chance of atlanto-axial subluxation. This presents as torticollis usually after 1–2 weeks.

Tonsillectomy

Common method used is dissection and snare method. Other methods are:

a. Cold methods

1. Dissection and snare
2. Guillotine (not used now)
3. Intracapsular tonsillectomy with debrider
4. Harmonic scalpel
5. Plasma-mediated ablation method
6. Cryosurgical technique.

b. Hot methods

1. Electrocautery
2. Laser (CO_2 or KTP)
3. Coblation
4. Radiofrequency

Q: What are the indications for tonsillectomy?

Ans:

- Absolute indications:
    - Chronic tonsillitis:
      Recurrent infections of throat >7 in one year
      > 5/year for 2 consecutive years
      > 3/year for 3 consecutive years
    - Peritonsillar abscess (Quincy) interval tonsillectomy is done
    - Hypertrophy of tonsil causing obstructive sleep apnea syndrome (OSAS), dysphagia, speech problems
    - Suspicion of malignancy, in unilateral tonsillar enlargement
- Relative
    - Carriers of diphtheria and *Streptococcus* hemolyticus
    - Tonsillitis causing febrile seizures
    - Tonsillar infection causing secondary effects on other organs like rheumatic fever, acute glomerulonephritis, etc.
    - As part of other operations as in palatopharyngoplasty for OSAS, glossopharyngeal neurectomy, removal of styloid process (nontonsillar indications).

Indications for Unilateral Tonsillectomy

- As excision biopsy of tonsil to determine a possible malignancy
- As an approach in excision styloid process
- Tonsillolith, tonsillar cyst, and impacted FB tonsil
- In branchial fistula to remove the complete tract, one end of tract being in posterior tonsillar pillar.

Contraindications

Acute respiratory infection, epidemic of polio in the vicinity, hemoglobin less than 10%, bleeding disorders, uncontrolled systemic diseases like diabetes, hypertension, cardiac diseases.

Anesthesia: GA with endotracheal intubation is preferred. Can also be done under local anesthesia in cooperative patients.

Position: Rose's position (described in adenoidectomy).

Steps

- Mouth opened with mouth gag and tongue blade
- Tonsil held with Dennis brown tonsil holding forceps and pulled inferomedially
- Incision made over reflexion of mucous membrane from anterior tonsillar pillar to tonsil midway between upper pole and lower pole. Instrument used is Waugh's tonsil dissection forceps with teeth
- Using Mollison's tonsillar dissector-cum-pillar retractor, dissect tonsil from tonsillar bed until lower pole is reached
- Eve's tonsillar snare is passed around the lower pedicle and is closed. It crushes and cuts through the pedicle and the tonsil gets separated
- Pack kept in tonsillar fossa. Same done on opposite tonsil.
- After pack removal, bleeding points if present are ligated or cauterized.

Postoperative Care

Normal unaided respiration should be established before the patient leaves operation theater. Keep patient in comma position/ tonsil position (turned to one side head flexed to a lower level). Keep a watch on bleeding, swallowing, respiration and pulse. Ice cold feeds started on complete recovery from anesthesia. Antibiotics, analgesics started. Good oral hygiene should be maintained. Patient discharged 24–48 hours after surgery. Can resume duties after one week.

- Average blood loss during tonsillectomy is 50–80 mL.
- It is 80–120 mL in combined adenotonsillectomy.

Complications

- Immediate
  - *Due to anesthesia:* Aspiration, hypotension, cardiac arrest
  - *Due to surgery:*
    - *Primary hemorrhage:* Caused by recent infection, undected bleeding diathesis, poor technique. Controlled with pressure, electrocoagulation and ligatures
    - *Injury to neighboring structures:* Teeth, tonsillar pillar, uvula, soft palate, tongue.
- Intermediate
  - *Reactionary hemorrhage:* Occurs within a period of 24 hours dangerous complication.

  Reasons are:
  - Slippage of knot tied at the time of surgery
  - Rebound hypertension on recovery from general anesthesia causes blood vessels to open up and to bleed.

  Arrange blood if needed. Correct fluid and electrolyte imbalance if any. If any clots in the tonsillar fossa it should be removed (presence of clot prevents clipping action of superior constrictor muscle on vessels) if bleeding is not controlled ligation/electrocoagulation of bleeding vessels done under general anesthesia.

- Delayed:
  - *Secondary hemorrhage:* Seen between 5 and 10 postoperative day. Usually caused by infection. It is an emergency.

Treatment of secondary hemorrhage:

- Admit
- Broad spectrum intravenous antibiotics
- Transfusion of blood or plasma depending on blood loss
- For profuse bleeding, ligature or electrocauterization of bleeding vessel under general anesthesia is needed. Bleeding if not controlled by this, approximation of pillares with mattress sutures or even external carotid artery ligation is needed.
  - Lung complications
  - Infection
  - Scarring of soft palate and pillars
  - Tonsillar remnants
  - Hypertrophy of lingual tonsil.
- Direct laryngoscopy, esophagoscopy and bronchoscopy dealt along with instruments.

CHAPTER 6

Objective Structured Clinical Examination

Many universities keep stations of objective structured clinical examination (OSCE) in practical examinations. It can be spotter, X-ray, instrument, audiograms or observer supervised stations for various procedures. The list is very vast. Commonly asked questions are included here:

SPOTTERS

Identify (Fig. 6.1)

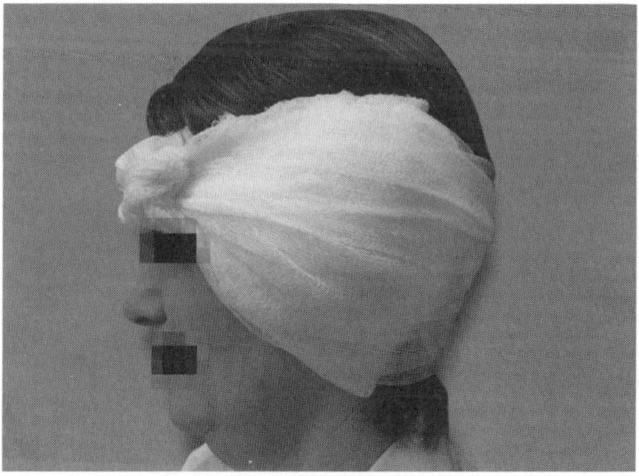

Fig. 6.1 Mastoid dressing

Ans: Patient (male/female) **(Fig. 6.1)** with mastoid dressing (right side).

Q1. Enumerate the indications.

Ans:

- Surgeries on mastoid
- Surgeries on pinna of ear (excision dermoid cyst, ceroma pinna)
- After cleaning/suturing pinna injuries/perichondritis pinna
- After surgeries on pre/postaural area (preauricular sinus excision).

Q2. Write indications/contraindications/complications of mastoid surgeries.

Ans: Given under operative surgery.

Q3. Name groups of mastoid air cells.

Ans: Nine groups—1. Mastoid antrum (largest and most constant air cell), 2. Petrous, 3. Perisinus, 4. Perilabyrinthine, 5. Peritubal, 6. Retrofacial, 7. Zygomatic, 8. Tip cells, 9. squamosal cells.

Q4. Name the parts of facial nerve.

Ans:

- Intracranial part
- Intratemporal part: (a) Meatal segment (b) Labyrinthine segment (c) Tympanic/horizontal segment (d) Mastoid/vertical segment
- Extracranial part.

Q5. What is facial recess? Describe its boundaries and surgical importance.

Ans: Space in the middle ear bounded by the facial nerve medially, laterally by chorda tympani, and superiorly by fossa incudis. Through this space middle ear can be accessed from the mastoid aspect. This is the surgical approach for cochlear implantation.

Q6. Name the abscesses in relation to mastoid diseases.

Ans:

- Postaural abscess—most common

- Zygomatic abscess
- Bezold abscess
- Meatal/Luc's abscess
- Citelli's abscess
- Parapharyngeal/retropharyngeal abscess.

Q7: List the complications of chronic suppurative otitis media) CSOM).

Ans:

- *Intratemporal/extracranial:*
  - Mastoiditis (most common complication) and mastoid abscess
  - Petrositis (Gradenigo's syndrome consisting of 3Ds discharge, deep-seated orbital pain (due to trigeminal neuralgia) and diplopia (lateral rectus palsy due to abducent nerve involvement)
  - Facial palsy
  - Labyrinthitis/labyrinthine fistula.
- *Intracranial:*
  - Extradural abscess
  - Subdural abscess
  - Brain abscess—the most common intracranial complication
  - Meningitis
  - Lateral sinus thrombosis
  - Otitic hydrocephalus.

Q8. What is Macewen's triangle? Define its boundaries and significance.

Ans: See operative surgery.

Q9. Name triangle in relation to temporal bone.

Ans:

- Macewen's
- Trautmann's.

Q10. Angles in relation to temporal bone.

Ans:

- Citelli's angle
- Antrum threshold angle
- Solid angle/hard angle.

Q11. What is Körner's septum?

Ans: See operative surgery.

Identify (Fig. 6.2)

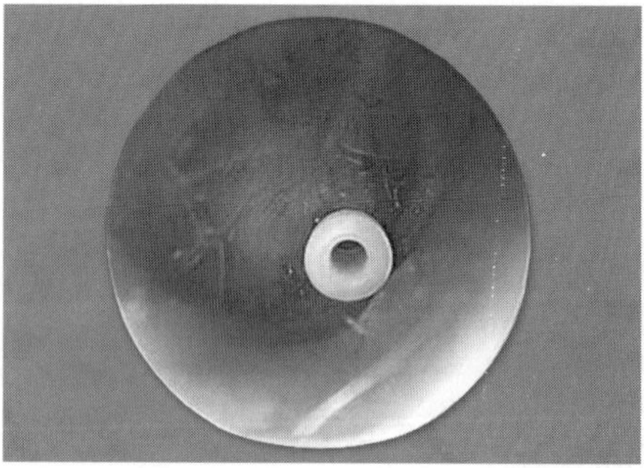

Fig. 6.2 Right tympanic membrane with ventilation tube in situ

Ans: Right tympanic membrane **(Fig. 6.2)** with ventilation tube in situ.

Q1. What is the purpose of putting ventilation tubes in suppurative otitis media (SOM)?

Ans: Ventilation tubes establish adequate aeration of middle ear cleft, with consequent reversion of pathological changes of middle ear mucosa.

Q2. Name some ventilation tubes.

Ans: Short-term: Shepard VT

Medium-term: Shah, Paparella, Armstrong

Long-term: Per-Lee, Goode T-tube.

Q3. Describe the indications of myringotomy, types of myringotomy and complications of myringotomy.

Ans: See operative surgery.

Q4. Medical treatment of otitis media with effusion (OME).

Ans: Antiallergic, steroids, decongestants, mucolytics and antibiotics (is of doubtful benefit).

Q5. What is the treatment of choice for otitis media with effusion (OME)?

Ans: Surgical—Myringotomy with VT insertion.

Q6. Name the four synonyms of OME.

Ans:

- Glue ear
- Otitis media with effusion
- Mucoid otitis media
- Serous otitis media.

Q7. The most common cause in children.

Ans: Allergy and adenoid hypertrophy.

Identify (Fig. 6.3)

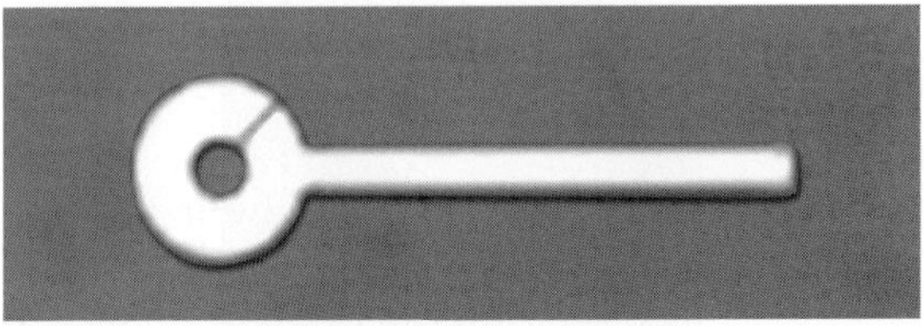

Fig. 6.3 Stapes piston

Ans: Stapes piston.

Q1. Write the uses.

Ans: Used in stapedectomy/stapedotomy (treatment of choice in otosclerosis).

Q2. What are the indications for stapedectomy?

Ans: Given under operative surgery—stapedectomy.

- Stapes piston made of Teflon is common.

Q3. What is the common clinical presentation of otosclerosis?

Ans: Painless and progressive bilateral conductive hearing loss usually starts in late 20s, more in females.

Q4: Typical PTA finding in otosclerosis.

Ans: Carhart's notch—dip at 2000 Hz in bone conduction.

Q5: Other treatment options.

Ans: Hearing aid.

Q6: What is the role of medicines?

Ans: No definite role. Sodium fluoride has been tried to hasten maturity of active focus and to arrest further cochlear damage.

Identify (Fig. 6.4)

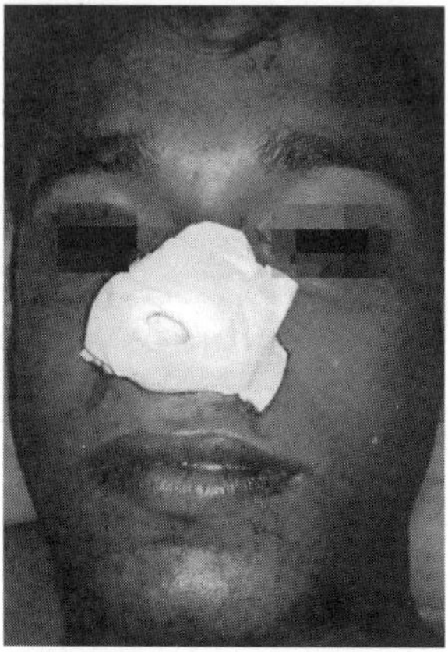

Fig. 6.4 Anterior nasal pack

Ans: Patient **(Fig. 6.4)** with anterior nasal pack in situ.

Identify (Fig. 6.5)

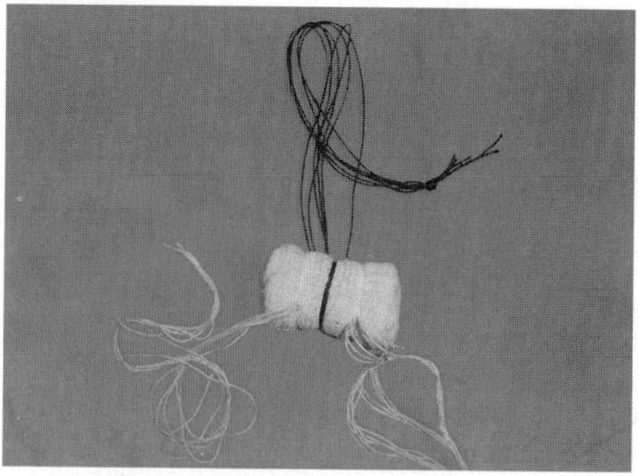

Fig. 6.5 Postnasal pack

Ans: Postnasal pack (**Fig. 6.5**).

Has one black thread and two white threads.

Q1. Describe the indications of nasal packing.

Ans:

- Epistaxis not controlled with pressure application
- After nasal surgeries such as septoplasty, SMR, endoscopic sinus surgery
- After drainage of septal abscess/hematoma.

Q2. Name the four local and four systemic causes of epistaxis.

Ans: Local causes: 1. Trauma; 2. Atrophic rhinitis; 3. Rhinolith; 4. Rhinosporidiosis nose.

Systemic causes: 1. Hypertension; 2. Liver disease like hepatic cirrhosis; 3. Kidney disease like chronic nephritis; 4. Drugs like anticoagulants.

Q3. What is little's area?

Ans: Area in the anteroinferior part of nasal septum. The most common site of epistaxis in children and young adults.

Q4. Name the arteries anastomosing in Little's area.

Ans: Four arteries—1. Anterior ethmoidal artery; 2. Septal branch of superior labial; 3. Septal branch of sphenopalatine artery; 4. Septal branch of greater palatine artery.

This anastomosis is called Kiesselbach's plexus.

Q5. What is Woodruff's area?

Ans: Arterial anastomotic area seen under the posterior end of inferior turbinate. Site of posterior epistaxis. Common site of bleeding in old age.

Q6. What are the methods to stop bleeding?

1. Anterior nasal/postnasal packing
2. Endoscopic sphenopalatine artery ligation (ESPAL)
3. Endoscopic cauterization
4. *Ligation of vessels:* External carotid artery, maxillary artery, Ethmoidal arteries.

Identify (Fig. 6.6)

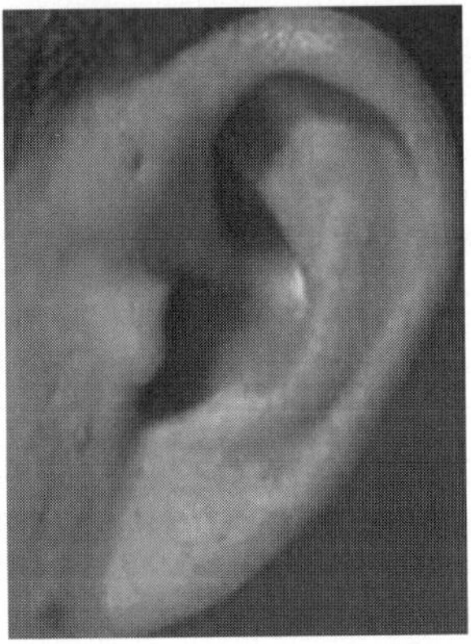

Fig. 6.6 Preauricular sinus

Ans: Preauricular sinus **(Fig. 6.6)** left side.

Developmental anomaly—faulty union of hillocks of 1st and 2nd branchial arches.

Treatment is complete excision. If not adequately treated chance of preauricular abscess or unsightly scar.

- *Collaural fistula*: Communication between external canal and neck. Caused by incomplete resorption of ventral portion of 1st branchial cleft.

Patient with LMN Facial Palsy

Q1. Define Bell's palsy.

Ans: Idiopathic peripheral facial paralysis or paresis of acute onset.

Q2. Define its treatment.

Ans:

1. *General:* Reassurance, care of eye, physiotherapy
2. *Medical:* Steroids-adult dose of prednisolone 1 mg/kg/day in divided dose tapered in 20 days. Along with this give vasodilators, vitamins, and symptomatic treatment.
3. *Surgery:* Nerve decompression relieves pressure on nerve fibers and improves microcirculation of the nerve.

Instruments, X-ray or audiograms can be kept as spotters.

Procedures that can be asked to perform in observer station

1. Any one of the tuning fork tests; 2. Fistula test; 3. Tragal sign; 4. Mastoid tenderness; 5. Nystagmus elicitation, etc.

AUDIOGRAMS

Symbols on audiogram (Fig. 6.7): Red represents right ear. Left ear marked with blue ink.

- *Pure tone:* Single frequency sound is called a *pure tone*. For example, sound of 250, 500 or 1000 Hz.
- *Decibel:* Named after Alexander Graham Bell, it is 1/10th of a bell. It is not an absolute figure. It represents a logarithmic ratio between two sounds.

	Right	Left
AC unmasked	○	×
AC masked	Δ	□
BC unmasked	<	>
BC masked	[	]
No response	↙	↘

Fig. 6.7 Symbols on audiogram

- *Noise:* A periodic complex sound
- *White noise:* It contains all frequencies in audible spectrum. This broadband noise is used for masking.
- *Masking:* It is a phenomenon to produce inaudibility of one sound by presentation of another.

Assessment of hearing: By clinical and audiometric tests,

- *Clinical tests of hearing:*
  - Finger friction test
  - Watch test
  - Speech test
  - Tuning fork tests.
- *Audiometric tests:*
  - Pure tone audiometry
  - Speech audiometry
  - Békésy audiometry
  - Impedence audiometry.

Pure Tone Audiogram (PTA)

Uses

- Used to record type and degree of hearing loss
- Used for documentation
- To find out degree of disability for medicolegal purpose
- To compare preoperative hearing level with that of postoperative results.

Normal Pure Tone Audiogram (Fig. 6.8) (Both Right and Left Sides)

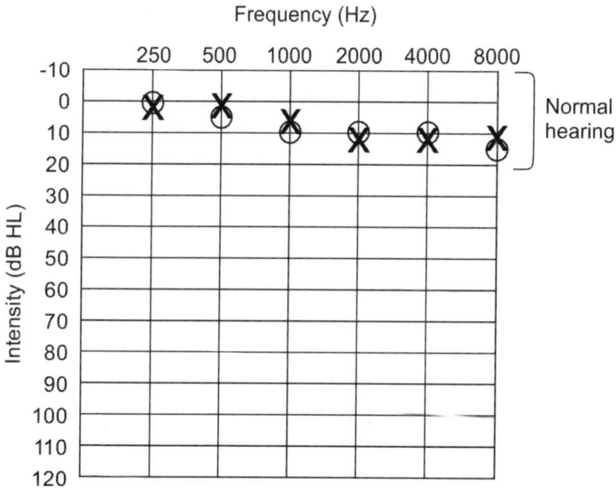

Fig. 6.8 Normal pure tone audiogram

Here, graph represents:

X-axis : Frequency in Hertz

Y-axis : Hearing loss in decibel

Ideally, AC and BC should overlap at 0 db. A gap of 10 dB is considered to be normal as there can be calibration difference of audiometer.

PTA of Conductive Hearing Loss (Right Side) (Fig. 6.9)

Here bone conduction thresholds are normal, but AC threshold has been increased with Air-Bone gap. This is typical of conductive hearing loss. Conductive hearing loss is caused by diseases of external ear or middle ear.

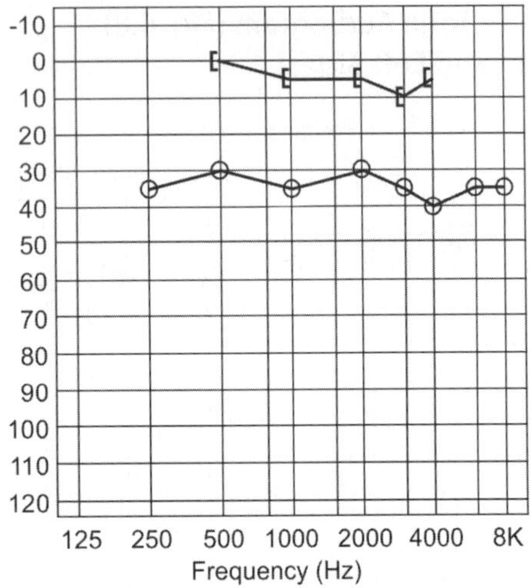

Fig. 6.9 PTA of conductive hearing loss

PTA of Sensorineural Hearing Loss (Both Ears) (Fig. 6.10)

Both AC and BC thresholds are increased with *no A-B gap.*

PTA of Mixed Hearing Loss (Fig. 6.11)

Both AC and BC thresholds increased and also there is *A-B gap.*

PTA of Noise-induced Hearing Loss (Fig. 6.12)

A *dip of air conduction at 4000 Hz* (Acoustic dip/Boiler Maker's notch) seen in NIHL.

PTA of Otosclerosis (Fig. 6.13)

Dip of bone conduction at 2000 Hz seen in otosclerosis. It is called *Carhart's notch.*

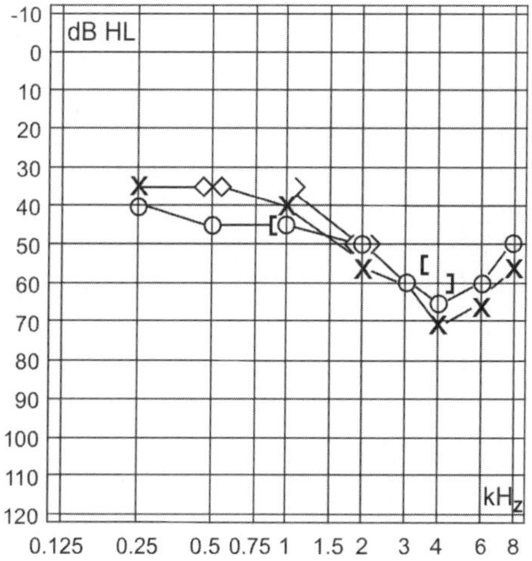

Fig. 6.10 PTA of sensorineural hearing loss

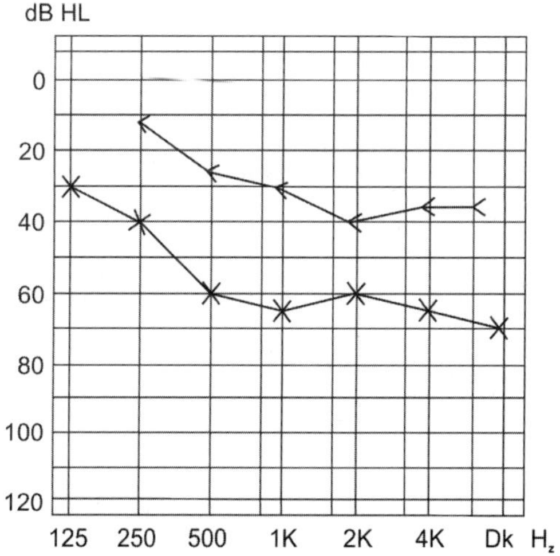

Fig. 6.11 PTA of mixed hearing loss

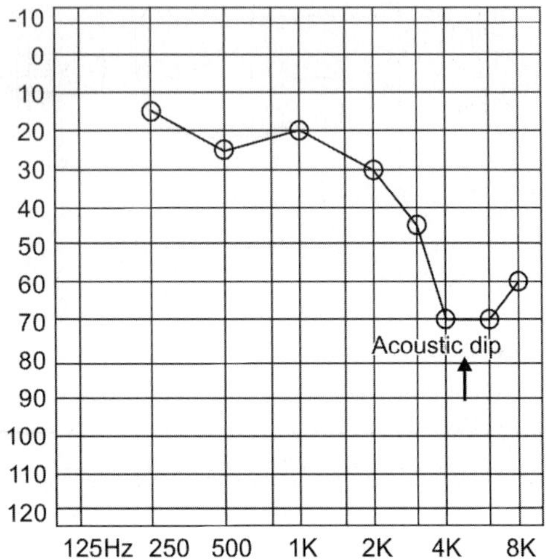

Fig. 6.12 PTA of noise-induced hearing loss

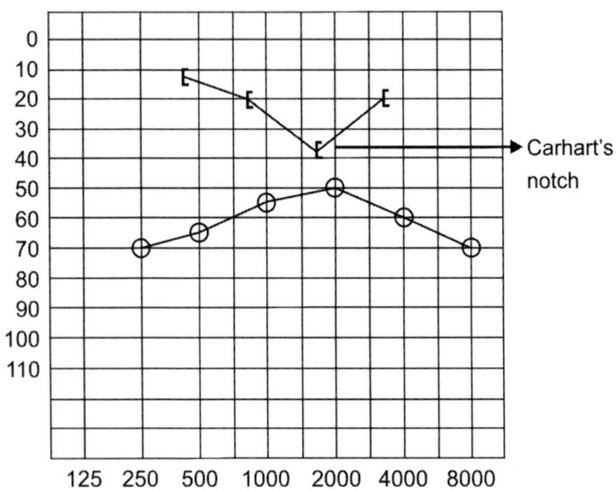

Fig. 6.13 PTA of otosclerosis

PTA of Congenital Deafness (Fig. 6.14)

Trough shaped (U-shaped/Basin-shaped) audiogram is seen in congenital deafness.

Q1. Name five anomalies of inner ear which can cause congenital hearing loss.

Ans:

1. Scheibe dysplasia
2. Alexander dysplasia
3. Bing-Siebenmann dysplasia
4. Michel dysplasia
5. Mondini dysplasia.

Q2. Name three syndromes associated with hearing loss.

Ans:

1. Waardenburg's syndrome
2. Pendred syndrome
3. Alport syndrome.

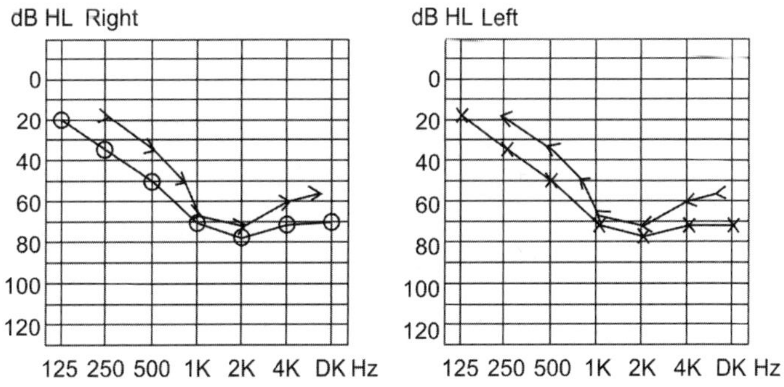

Fig. 6.14 PTA of congenital deafness

PTA of Presbyacusis and Ménière's Disease along with Tympanograms (Figs 6.15 to 6.18)

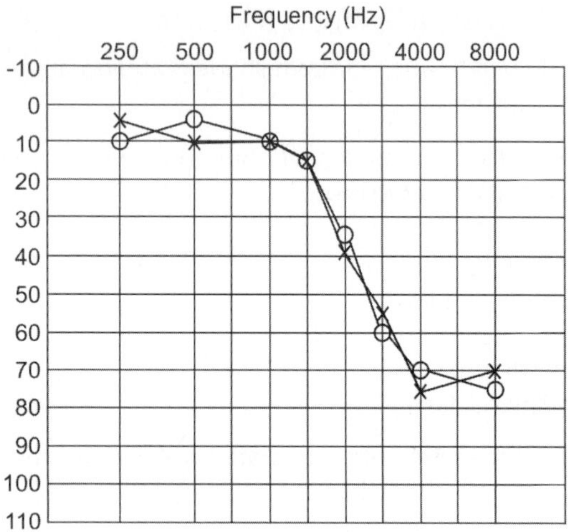

Fig. 6.15 PTA of presbyacusis

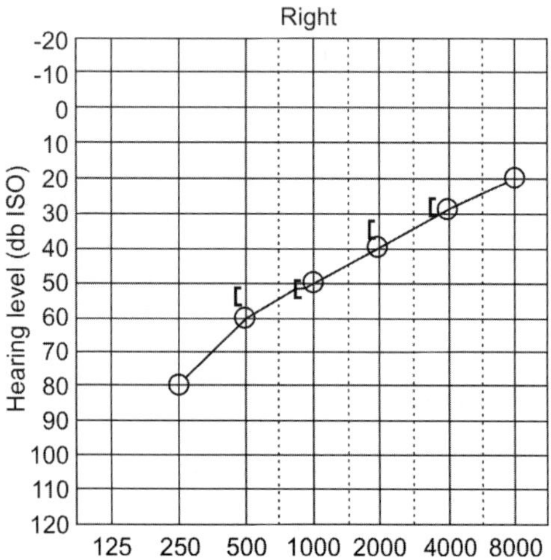

Fig. 6.16 PTA of Ménière's disease

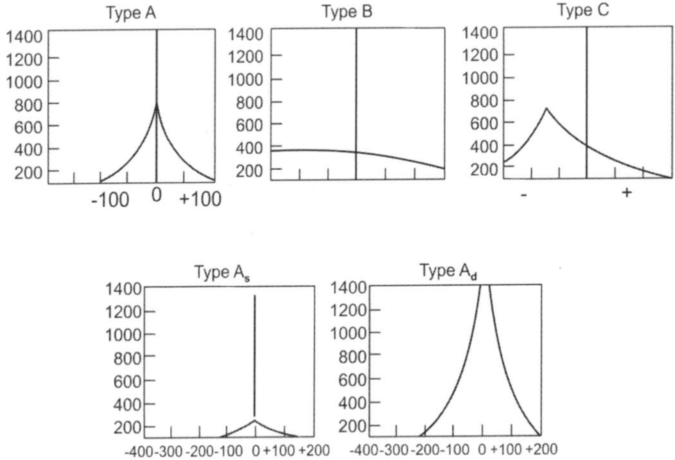

Fig. 6.17 Tympanograms

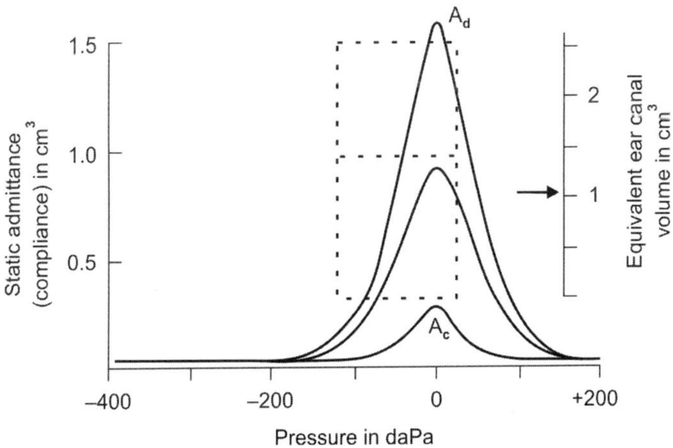

Fig. 6.18 Tympanogram

PTA of Presbyacusis (Fig. 6.15)

Bilateral high frequency sensorineural hearing loss. Low frequencies are relatively normal.

PTA of Ménière's Disease (Fig. 6.16)

Low frequency SN hearing loss.

Tympanogram (Figs 6.17 and 6.18)

It is the impedence audiogram. Measure of pressure of middle ear in X-axis and compliance (mobility) of tympano-ossicular system in Y-axis. Commonly, we get five types of curves:

A: Normal

A_s: Reduced compliance at normal pressure. Seen in otosclerosis, tympanosclerosis, ossicular fixity.

A_d: Very high compliance and normal pressure. Ossicular discontinuity/Lax TM

B: Flat curve. Typical of fluid in middle ear in SOM. Also seen in perforated TM.

C: Maximum compliance at negative pressure. Seen in eustachian tube dysfunction.

Index

Page numbers followed by *f* refer to figure

A

B

C

D

E

F

G

H

I

J

K

L

M

N

O

P

R

S

T